A Doctor's Guide to
Transform Your Pain to Pearls of Wisdom and Joy

U R NOT
WHAT U EAT

DR ZVI PEARLSTEIN

Contents

1

My Search for Answers

M y mother, Celia, who passed on in August 2019, was a Holocaust survivor from Poland. She experienced untold horrors as a teenager and the resulting emotional pain lived on with her throughout her life. Her pain was the source of many heartfelt writings and poetry about her experiences. I absorbed her pain in the womb, and from as early as I can remember, life for me became a search for answers to understand, explain, and solve that pain.

My father, Norman, who passed on in October 2018, had his own share of pain. He grew up in poverty. His parents escaped the pogroms of Russia at a young age and his father had a crippling stroke at the age of forty. The recent passing of both of my parents is the immediate impetus for me to write this book in their memory and merit.

My life has always been a search for answers and meaning, especially to unravel my identity and to make sense of it, amidst so much pain. I assumed that doing and achieving the best I could would take me to the places I needed to be to find what I was seeking. For the first seventeen years of my life I was a high achiever in academics, music, and sports. That got me to Princeton University where I spent four years obtaining my BA in biochemistry. Then, not completely sure if I wanted to attend medical school, I deferred my acceptance to New York University School of Medicine for one year during which I worked in a variety of jobs including as a tennis instructor, water analysis chemist, and musician. During that year, while living in Florida, I took my oath of office at Homestead Air Force Base, joining the United States Air Force as part of a scholarship program to pay for medical school. I went through basic training for offi-cers that year. I also visited Israel.

My search continued at New York University School of Medicine for four years while obtaining my MD. Then at State University of New York at Downstate in Brooklyn for five years while pursuing my orthopedic surgery residency. Then three years serving as a Major practicing ortho-pedic surgery with the United States Air Force overseas at Clark Air Base in the Philippines. I also helped man clinics and set up portable hospitals in Okinawa, South Korea, Japan, China, Guam, and the Azores. Then I spent a year doing orthopedic surgery at Andrews Air Force Base in Wash DC where I was an assistant professor at the Uniformed Services Health Science Center in Bethesda, MD. Subsequently I was called up and re-ported for active duty wartime service during Persian Gulf I.

Up to this point my life had been a search and journey spanning thir-ty-five years. It was mostly a subconscious endeavor and I don't know that I could have verbalized my life's mission or purpose then. Even though I did not know what I was searching for, I assumed that by seeking the highest level of achievement, I would find life's greatest and most profound meaning and answers. But the deep answers I yearned for and needed for so long were not forthcoming- not from my beloved parents or other family members, my friends, my teachers and professors, my varied experiences, or from anywhere I looked. Though others with whom I crossed paths along the way were content with what they had learned and what they were able to accomplish, I did not find what I was searching for and I was far from content. Through all of that hard work, and despite a very high level of accomplishment, I was left empty.

After my service in the Air Force, I married and began working as an orthopedic surgeon in Orange County, California. With a wife, good career, good income, nice home, and with hobbies in which I had advanced skills including playing trumpet and tennis, I imagine that I had everything anyone could wish for. Finally, I had reached the place that my endeavors and search had led me to, and one might think that I would have been very thankful and happy. But I was suddenly stricken by a deep sense of emptiness and depression.

Although I was successful at each endeavor I undertook, ultimately the mission statement of finding answers to my mother's pain, life's pain, and my life's questions was not fulfilled. I had gone to the pinnacles of learning, understanding, and challenges that existed as far as I knew, and I didn't know where else to go. I didn't sense that there was anyplace else to look.

My senior associate, who I had joined in his orthopedic surgery practice in southern California, was a Holocaust survivor from Hungary who had been in the Buchenwald concentration camp. His story, his accent, and his life apart from orthopedics, were very familiar to me. I joined him as a reminder of my mother's experience and pain, of all the Holocaust survivors I had known, and of my life's mission to search out life's ultimate answers. To make my task more pressing, not only was I depressed during much of the time that I worked in that practice, but many if not most of my patients also seemed to be depressed.

My patients had complaints of physical pain, but more often than not, their pain seemed to originate in a nonphysical source rather than a physical one. The more I spoke with the patients, the more I learned of their painful loneliness, relationship abuse, and pain involving spouse, parents, and children. There were social, work, financial, and other problems and abuses. This was an unexpected and unusual experience for me. I sensed that if I could find a solution with answers to my life, these same answers might be helpful to many of my patients.

The practice of orthopedic surgery usually does not lend itself to lengthy history taking and deep understanding of patients' life issues and how these relate to their pain. Ordinarily, it is not difficult for an orthopedic surgeon to turn back, neck, knee, shoulder and other pains into surgeries. But I was on a quest and needed answers and therefore spent hours conversing with patients. I was essentially conducting my own research study to find "the truth."

Whereas up to this point my quest for answers to pain was primarily about my Mom and me, it suddenly became also about my patients in pain who were presenting to me as their orthopedic surgeon, seeking and expecting answers from me. They generally expected a quick-fix surgical solution. But there were so many patients who in my opinion did not require a surgical solution or even any particular medical one. These patients were complaining of physical pain, but on very lengthy evaluation, I determined that the source of their pain was nonphysical life issues. Up till then I had practiced in settings where the typical orthopedic patient was physically "damaged" and required "fixing."

Finding many patients whose pain seemed to derive from their life issues rather than physical damage was a startling discovery for me. Never during my orthopedic training, nor during my practice from medical school and residency through my experience in the military, had I ever been exposed to the possibility that many patients presenting with orthopedic complaints might be manifesting bodily pain, however, the true source of their pain might be found in nonphysical sources. I felt all alone in my discovery and I knew of no one in orthopedic surgery to whom I could turn to share my experiences. By this time, my search for answers and understanding of pain was deeply intertwined with solving my patients' pain.

One day during this time that I was seeking answers yet feeling confused and depressed, a younger cousin who was also living in Southern California asked me if I wanted free tickets that he had to a Chabad (acronym for chochmah, binah, and daas or knowledge, wisdom, and understanding in Hebrew) Lubavitch (luba=love and vitch=city, city of love in Russia) fundraiser for Russian Jewry. I had no idea what this was about, but I accepted the tickets. My wife and I went to this function at the Wilshire Ebell Theater in Los Angeles. The event turned out to be awesomely transformative for me.

The first thing that blew me away was a video presentation that showed Russian Jews who had been deprived in Russia of the ability to live as practicing Jews. Suddenly they were excited, joyous, and thrilled to experience Jewish life. The video showed Russians undergoing circumcision, bar mitzvah, praying, going to synagogue, lighting a Chanuka menorah, kissing a mezuzah (parchment-filled case on doorposts), putting on tefillin (parchment-filled black boxes with attached straps that are worn by men on the head and left upper arm next to the heart during weekday prayer) and tzitzis (men's shirt undergarment with attached strings that serves as a reminder of the 613 mitzvahs of the Jewish bible known as the Torah). They were celebrating Shabbos (Jewish Sabbath) and the Jewish holidays of Rosh Hashana, Yom Kippur, Sukkos, Pesach, Shavuos, Chanuka, Purim.

As I watched, I couldn't help but wonder why when all my life I was not living in communist Russia, but had been living free in America, the joyous experience of these mitzvahs (the 613 commandments of the Torah also known as good deeds or connections to G0d (this altered spelling will be used throughout this book as a show of respect and humility) or actions of lovingkindness in all our relationships including with others, G0d, ourselves, and animals, plants, and the material world) was not part of my life. I knew why Russian Jews were prevented from living a religious life, but I questioned why this lifestyle with these mitzvahs and the associated joy were not part of my life and why I had never been properly educated in their practice?

My whole life all I knew was the pain of being a Jew and the pain of Judaism. My mother survived the Holocaust and my father's parents escaped the pogroms in Russia, and all my parents' friends that I was exposed to in my childhood were Holocaust survivors. The burden of bearing this painful history and heritage was excruciating. Why was I deprived, like these Russian Jews, of the joy of Judaism? Why was my identity a pile of pain when it could have been a solid foundation of time-honored joyful practices?

All of a sudden, the level of joy at the event rose several notches when several well-known singers performed. These included Rabbi Salzman, a very special bald-headed chazan (religious Jewish singer) from Russia, and Moshe Yess, the rock and roll singer guitarist who became religiously involved later in life and is best known for his wonderfully special simultaneously tearful and joyful song, My Zaidi (grandfather). While the singing was going on, a group of men in long black coats with beards and black hats jumped on stage. Becoming very light of foot they jumped and danced causing the level of joy I was experiencing to be magnified.

In all my thirty-five years of life, this was my first exposure to the joy of Judaism. I had tears of joy and chills of excitement. Suddenly, steeped in my own personal pain and depression, I was given a window to the possibility of answers to what ailed me for so long. This was the first moment and first day in my next journey, a thirty-year journey till now, and an ongoing lifelong journey experiencing the fulfilling life of a practicing and learning Jew.

For much of my life to that point, I was repeatedly told that I was not a "team player." I didn't really know what that meant because I thought I was always trying to do the right thing. Eventually when I fortuitously "bumped" into G0d and the struggle-filled journey of establishing my own identity as Divine Soul (Since the Soul and the Divine or G0dly Soul refer to a piece of G0d that resides equally in all humankind, I have decided to capitalize Soul and Divine Soul throughout this book), I finally figured it out. Whether at Princeton University, New York University School of Medicine, SUNY Downstate, the United States Air Force, or in various practices, the people in power were generally expecting me to "bow down" to the same gods they had accepted for themselves. I might not have known enough about G0d yet, but I did have enough intuitive sense to know that I would not accept their gods or their belief systems.

I learned what I had to learn that was true and ignored or discarded what did not make sense to me. Spurred on by my deep connection with my mother's pain, I needed more. I needed the ultimate true answers and not just the popular temporary fixes that many people settle for. I needed the Truth. It was not until I discovered the path to develop my identity as Divine Soul and learned to actualize my life based on that identity, and learned a way to connect with G0d, that I found the "team" I had always been searching for. Suddenly, for the first time in my life, being a team player became natural. Unbeknownst to me, I had always been searching for the ultimate team-G0d's team. I finally found my team.

I was aware from a young age of the importance to pursue academic pursuits for mind development and physical fitness and exercise for bodily health. I was living the familiar mind and body paradigm and was sure that pursuing a career in medicine would keep my mind strong and my gym workouts, tennis, running, and my generally active lifestyle would keep my body healthy. The concept of Soul was previously not part of my health paradigm and was probably not even part of my consciousness. Becoming aware of a new way of understanding myself and humankind, after so many years of thinking I was on the right track, was startling for me. Suddenly, I was awakened and life took on a fresh and new beginning. I was reborn.

My long journey of searching brought me first to orthopedics as my career and profession. Later on, my journey brought me to authentic Judaism where I encountered the word "orthodox." How unusual that I should end up confronting a word that was so similar to the name for my medical specialty. "Ortho" means straight and "pedics" means children. Orthopedics etymologically essentially means to help children grow physically straight. The word itself has no etymological connection to muscle, bones, joints, tendons, or ligaments. Orthopedics could have been the term for all of physical medicine and the medical science involved with promoting all of bodily healing.

It is truly ironic that the word for my physical career work and the word connected to my spiritual work are so similar. One might mistakenly think that orthodox is an abbreviation for orthopedic doctors. "Ortho" once again means straight and "dox" means doctrine. Doctrine refers to matters of the Soul, intellect, and emotions. Orthodox etymologically essentially means to help children grow nonphysically or spiritually straight.

As a practicing orthopedic surgeon for many years, becoming familiar, learning, and practicing authentic Judaism with its "orthodoxy" caused a huge dilemma for me. Basic to Judaism are concepts of G0d and Soul. In orthopedics, medicine, and healthcare delivery generally, G0d and Soul have been traditionally non-existent and unacceptable concepts. Practitioners are often ready to dismiss and frown on these terms as well as on those people who might use them. The dilemma and challenge I suddenly faced was that if I accepted as true the foundational premises in Judaism of G0d and Soul, then the practice of orthopedic surgery and medicine, despite much so good work, promotes a false belief system.

Without a concept of Soul, instead of doing what one might think healthcare is meant to do-help us to achieve wholeness-it can do exactly the opposite and turn us into but a small fraction of our true selves. We can be readily reduced by the healthcare system to an identity consisting of just a body, or merely diseased body parts, or a single diseased body part. Without a concept of one G0d and faith in one G0d, an infinite number of false gods can be fashioned in the healthcare system including doctors, technologies, X-rays, MRI's, medications, procedures, surgeries, hospitals, profit motive, and much more. I concluded that fostering healing, wholeness, and hope, and avoidance of unnecessary and inappropriate reliance on and utilization of medical services would be optimally achieved only by incorporation of the concepts of G0d and Soul in the practice of medicine and the healthcare system.

My discovery excited me, and I was sure I was not the first one to have experienced this transformation and revelation. Those who had traveled a similar path to me, I assumed, must have already established somewhere a broader practice of medicine incorporating concepts of G0d and Soul. I was enthusiastic to find and join this G0d and Soul based medicine wherever it was. Surely then my dilemma would be solved. But I searched and searched yet did not find what I was looking for.

Although rare individual doctors might selectively incorporate the concepts of G0d and Soul in their practice, and others have written critically of our healthcare system, I could find no system of medicine applying these concepts. Faith-based medicine does outreach with religious organizations, but I have not found a faith-based system of medical practice incorporating concepts of G0d and Soul. Thomas Moore and others like him have written on the Soul and its relevance in healthcare, however, he is a psychotherapist and author, not a physician.

The physician and surgeon who I found myself to be most aligned with in thinking, writing, and practice is Dr. Bernie Siegel, the author of the precious book "Love, Medicine and Miracles." I have read his books, heard him lecture, met him, and interviewed him on a radio show I had. Dr. Siegel's writings and teachings make a beautiful and wonderful bridge between Soul and body. He has been impactful on the lives of so many, especially with his very helpful treatment paradigms for women with breast cancer and his Exceptional Cancer Patients (ECP) non-profit organization. He is known for establishing the concept that the morbidity and mortality of breast cancer patients is dramatically reduced when the disease is handled by a group of affected women rather than individually. However, I am unaware of a system of medicine or medical entity incorporating Dr. Siegel's amazing concepts and work regarding the relationship of Soul and body.

The nearest I came to find a solution in an organization that I might be able to join is GWISH based at George Washington University in Wash DC. GWISH stands for George Washington Institute for Spirituality and Health. The founder and director of GWISH, Dr. Christina Puchalski, who is an internist, does an amazing job of introducing spiritual depth to the practice of medicine. However, as wonderful as she and her program are, to my disappointment, last I checked, their scope is limited primarily to the arena of death and dying. In the paradigm that I find truthful, G0d and Soul don't just show up at the end of life. They are involved in all of life. I needed more.

More:

There are several messages from G0d in the Torah regarding the source of healing and health. For example, *"If you obey G-d your L0ʳᵈ and do what is upright in His eyes, carefully heeding all His Commandments and keeping all His decrees, then I will not strike you with any of the sicknesses that I brought on Egypt. I am the G-d Who heals you."* (Ex. 15:23-25) If G0d is the true healer, then certainly we have to give Him credence when entertaining health and healing.

When corporate Home Depot gave me the opportunity to create a network of clinics providing work comp services for their southern California stores, I visited clinics to recruit them. The first thing the clinic owners wanted to know was, "Are you going to get more MRI's and make more surgeries?" I told them that we would acquire more patients from Home Depot and a variety of other home service stores, but that I did not expect the number of MRI's or surgeries to increase. That was not an adequate answer for them. They wanted to hear that more MRI's and subsequent surgeries would be done.

Because of my beard and religious appearance at the time, as well as my philosophy of care, they warned me not to bring any talk of G0d, soul, or religious concepts into their clinics. They all were vehement that healthcare and concepts relegated to religion do not mix. One of the clinic owners was somewhat more lenient and told me he would have no problem incorporating religious teaching and lessons into patient care, so long as we could get paid for it. Although Home Depot made me a wonderful offer, I was idealistic in my goals and I could not come to terms with any clinics to deliver my paradigm of care. As we commonly find in American healthcare, the bottom line for the clinics was not patient welfare and wellness, but instead was profit motive.

2

The Half-Shekel Paradigm

D uring the first year of my new life at age thirty-five, I ran into a concept that overwhelmed me. According to the Torah, when the Jews were wandering in the desert after having received the Torah at Mount Sinai, they were commanded by G0d to have a Mishkan (Tabernacle or synagogue-like place of worship) with them at all times. In order to build the Mishkan, G0d told Moshe (Moses, meaning drawn from the water) that every Jew had to contribute one half-shekel (Israeli coin with minimal value) towards the construction project. Moshe didn't initially comprehend G0d's request. He asked G0d why someone with great wealth couldn't contribute more and why someone who had nothing at all nevertheless had to contribute the half-shekel. G0d answered by throwing out His extended anthropomorphic arm and hand with palm up toward Moshe and in His palm was a fiery half-shekel.

The explanation for this encounter is that the Soul identity of each one of us is incomplete and on its own is at most half of a whole. To complete ourselves, the other half must come from G0d. As long as we are each willing to fulfill our responsibilities, to each connect our half-shekel to G0d, then G0d will partner fifty-fifty to allow each of us to find wholeness and peace. Further elaboration of the half-shekel concept is that all of our relationships and connections are optimally half-shekel relationships. These half-shekel or fifty-fifty relationships are about two halves coming together and connecting to make a whole, and ideally each participant is expected to contribute 100% effort.

A corollary to the half-shekel concept is that our identity is determined by the sum total of our connections and how we prioritize them. A huge key to a successful life is to choose our connections and relationships wisely and to prioritize them wisely. G0d never plays second fiddle, so a top priority for each one of us is to always work especially hard and be vigilant to strive to maintain our half-shekel relationship with G0d. G0d is and will always be there for us. It is up to us to do our part to recognize and connect with G0d. This is a powerful lesson for healing as well as living.

First and foremost, we have the ability to acknowledge and look to G0d as our Creator, as the source of all life and the source of all healing. As we gain wisdom, we can learn to understand the science of G0dly healing, which is an ongoing process of each of our cells, organs, and entire bodies. The more we understand, the better we can optimally utilize doctors, testing, medication, treatment, surgery, and hospital interventions to further promote the already present healing process and avoid unnecessary and inappropriate measures.

The balance between looking to G0d for healing and looking to doctors is easily clarified with the following example. If we scrape our skin, none of us run to the doctor, and we know the skin will heal. Yet no one can explain how the healing actually occurs. This process of healing is not actively controlled or monitored by our brains and no doctor is involved. The process is of the body, yet, like all bodily healing, it is empowered by the combination of energy from the Soul and energy from G0d. For optimal healing it is important to avoid abuse of the affected area. Complete healing with scab formation and skin remodeling might take one to two months.

If we now consider the very common and costly problem of low back pain which has been reported to approach $100 billion per year, people readily and often immediately run to many kinds of treatments, tests, devices, and surgeries. Surely if a scrape might require one to two months to heal completely, low back pain can be expected to take longer. Why do people irrationally expect healing of low back pain and other common muscle and joint ailments in a matter of a few days? Wisdom regarding the true process of healing is sorely lacking by the general public.

Science tells us that as we age, the water content of our tissues decreases on a cellular level and the tissues become less fluid with increasing stiffness. With aging we become less mobile and active and more sedentary. Over many years as our muscles and ligaments are moved less and less, they will tend to shorten, stiffen, and tighten to the point of maximum motion. The result of this process that commonly occurs concomitantly with aging is pain and stiffness.

The way we are made by G0d, regular full range of motion of our muscles and joints is a wonderful tool to prevent this problem of low back pain and many other muscle and joint pains. Avoidance of injury is of course also very important. Yet, once this pain exists people generally don't seem to recognize three important aspects of healing that are part of the science of G0dly healing. First, be careful not to overuse or abuse the body which can cause more harm. Second, gentle daily full range of motion of the affected muscle and joint grouping is not only the key to prevention, it is also the key to recovery. Third, healing occurs in G0d's time and not immediately by pressing a button.

People tend to have a push-button mentality and the desire for an immediate quick fix, coupled with a lack of wisdom about how the healing process truly works. The result is that patients often lack the patience required to allow the process of healing to progress to completion. Instead of allowing healing to occur over the required longer period of time than they generally expect or desire, patients often readily opt for all kinds of procedures and surgeries. Patients and their treating doctors often don't allow adequate time for Soul and G0d directed healing. Instead, patients allow the doctors and their technologies to supplant the roles of Soul and God in healing thereby dismissing their associated healing power.

Many people have been conditioned to think that solutions to complicated problems can be as simple as pressing a tv control button. But low
back pain can be the result of forty, fifty, sixty, or more years of living.
To expect pain to resolve in a day or two or even within weeks may be
very unrealistic. In G0d's time, low back pain can take many weeks to
months to resolve with healthy care. Yet unlike the lack of fear people have
in self-treatment of scrapes of the skin, many people with low back pain
and other joint pains readily run to all types of doctors for all kinds of
treatments and surgeries of their backs and joints.

A greater awareness and understanding of the science of G0dly healing
combined with our current medical knowledge would go a long way to
improving healthcare. The public could be educated how to evaluate and
self-treat many problems and to triage ourselves with the knowledge of how
to distinguish the three types of problems we experience: emergencies that
require immediate care, urgent problems that are not life threatening but
need evaluation soon, and problems that with proper self-care and sometimes with a physician's guidance would likely improve and heal over time.

As early as thirty years ago, I felt a burning need to bridge the medical and orthopedic world with the world of G0d and Soul. Toward that
purpose, I had in mind and have repeatedly attempted to start a healthcare
company and have had many false starts. The challenge has made me
stronger and more determined. With the recent loss of my parents came
the greater recognition that life is short and that with the passing of every
day my time is more limited. So, I am at it again. Now that my dear father
is no longer here, I'd like to recognize and honor him for providing the
original name of this endeavor.

Thirty years ago, struck by the powerful meaning of the half-shekel
concept, I told my Dad that I wanted to name my company by a name
that meant half-shekel. He did not blink and responded immediately, "Call
it Halbeshekel." I asked him, "What is Halbeshekel?" He told me that
it was Yiddish (a language combining elements of Hebrew and German
that was spoken by Ashkenazic eastern European Jews) for half-shekel.
I thought my Dad's response was brilliant and I loved it. He always was

brilliant. Halbeshekel is a name that few would recognize as having any meaning, but that on taking a deeper look would be found to have profound meaning.

It was not even a year later that I was visiting my uncle and aunt in Israel that my uncle asked me if he'd ever shown me a four-volume series of books published in 1873 in Lemberg, Poland, which were written by my grandfather's relative of the same last name. To my astonishment these books were titled Machazit Hashekel in Hebrew which in English means Half-Shekel. The synchronicity of the name and the timing of this revelation served as a sign of confirmation for me that I was on the right track. My uncle endowed me with my own complete four-volume set of these books. I subsequently learned that these books written by my relative are part of accepted Jewish law.

Since my revelation and the beginning of my process of Soul Transformation thirty years ago, I have developed the concepts in this book as well as a variety of products, services, courses, books, e-books, videos, and inventions. I have held onto the name Halbeshekel for my company all this time since my father gifted me with it. Recently, though, in preparation for launching the company, out of nowhere the name Missing Links Health entered my brain.

Each time I have developed a new concept, product, service, or invention, when I subsequently researched and found that no one had already created something similar, I could not understand why not. All of my ideas and creations seemed like "missing links" to me. They should have already been created and on the market.

The name Missing Links Health additional relevance since a link is not unlike a joint in orthopedics. Also, Halbeshekel is all about making proper healthy connections beginning with a connection and relationship with G0d. Any missing essential connections in our lives might also be called "missing links." And so, we have come full circle in that Halbeshekel and Missing Links Health both convey the same meaning about the paramount importance of the connections we make in our lives.

Halbeshekel dba (doing business as) Missing Links Health is about providing novel, unique, better, and cost-saving health, wellness, and fitness solutions for people, patients, workers, businesses, and insurance companies. This category of business is known as healthcare disruption. The healthcare industries we disrupt are Diet and Weight Loss, Mental Health, Addiction and Recovery, Pain Management, Fitness and Exercise, Corporate and Organizational Wellness, Sedentary Disease, Alzheimer's Disease and Senile Dementia of aging, and MRI and Surgery.

In this book I draw from all my lessons and experiences as the son of a Holocaust survivor mother, and from family, academia, medicine, orthopedic surgery, religion, music, health, fitness, exercise, wellness lifestyle, sports, and life to offer up alternative answers and ways of understanding life. This process arose from learning to be skilled to use a scalpel as a surgeon yet knowing that relatively few people need the surgical skills of a surgeon for healing. More people need the physician for medical advice. Most people need the physician as a human being to hear about their problems.

All people seeking healing are dealing with a process that mandates a relationship with G0d, whether they recognize it or not. Through a process of learning, growth, and transformation, I became this doctor functioning always as a human being to hear the patient's problems and seeking to connect the patient and G0d for healing, always available as medical doctor to offer medical advice to educate and impart wisdom, and always available to do surgery when necessary. By providing a listening ear and wisdom education for patients, the need for surgery becomes greatly diminished.

The meaning, happiness, joy, wholeness, and peace I have subsequently found and have been graced with in my life results from applying much of what I have written here. In this book I share many of the concepts that I found helpful in my search to understand, combat, and conquer the pain I knew from my mother, that I experienced in my life, and that I helped my patients overcome. These concepts became the foundational principles of my life and of my company Halbeshekel dba Missing Links Health and its products and services.

I truly hope and pray that in the merit of both of my parents' lives as well as those that came before, in the merit of all the Holocaust survivors, in the merit of all those innocents whose lives were taken, in the merit of all those who have struggled with pain, and in the merit of the children and all of the innocent yet unborn lives, this book and my other related endeavors will help many of you to understand, combat, and conquer your pain. By doing so you can achieve a higher more meaningful and reward-ing state of joyful living with happiness and wholeness. Whether you are challenged by physical, emotional, or spiritual pain, or have lived through a hell like the Holocaust as did my mother, you can learn to be more than a survivor. You can overcome and thrive!

More:

When a patient presents with the complaint of a specific body part like pain of the low back, the assumption by the patient and generally by the treating doctors is that they need to address the low back. Often a lumbar MRI study and surgery are performed. That is because of their collective assumption that the cause of the complaint of low back pain is to be found in the low back and, more specifically, in whatever the radiologist's report of MRI images of the low back indicates. This assumption is sometimes true. But in my own life and in medical practice, I found that we humans are not as simple as "what you see is what you get."

"A book is not its cover" applies here and means that very often, pain can be much more complex than what doctors and the rest of us have been led to believe. For a patient and doctors to reduce the patient to being only low back pain, or their low back, or any other body part for that matter, and to the labels or diagnoses accompanying MRI results, is only useful in truly emergency or urgent situations. However, in most cases, there is much more to explore.

If all the physician knows and explores is the patient's complaint of low back pain, then low back pain is #1, and if the doctor you're seeing is a back surgeon, then doing back surgery is his #1, and low back surgery is a likely outcome. But if the physician were to dig deeper and discuss all the painful things in the patient's life, what if he finds that the most painful thing is their divorce, and the next most painful thing is their father recently passed away. Next is their bad financial situation, and next is their only child lives far away, and next is their car problems, and on and on, until we find that low back pain is not the #1 cause of pain in the patient's life, but instead is #10.

Perhaps the low back pain at #10 is merely a manifestation of the combination of #1-#9. We and the patient and the doctor will only know this if we know how important life issues are in determining the real source of any pain and are willing to search to identify and unravel these sources of pain. Skills for personal and medical clarification, understanding, and management of our life issues, and not just doctor visits, pills, MRI's, and surgeries, are extremely important for both patient and doctor to help prevent and recover from pain.

Another way of explaining this concept is with a simple story. One evening a man was taking a walk when he saw another man searching the ground for something. Upon inquiring what he was looking for, the man taking a walk and observing the other man was told that he was looking for his keys. The second man offered to help and immediately joined the search looking for the keys in the same location where the first man was searching. After considerable time passed without finding the keys, the passerby asked the other man where exactly he lost his keys. He pointed a short distance away to an area that did not include the location where they had been unsuccessfully searching for a long time. The passerby was disturbed and asked why they were not looking for the keys where they were lost. The owner of the keys told him that there was a streetlight where they were looking so certainly, they could see. Furthermore, it was too dark where he dropped his keys so they would never be able to find them there.

The point and relevance of this story is that learning brings light. But that learning and light are only relevant to a corresponding problem. Just because there is a certain light, it doesn't mean that's the place to look for a solution to a particular problem. In medicine, the wrong diagnosis, the wrong type of doctor for a specific problem, the wrong testing or interpretation of test results, the wrong understanding of the healing process are all examples of bringing the "wrong light" to bear on a problem.

Some concepts and "lights" apply to only certain circumstances in life. Practical examples of this are our job skills and medical specialty knowledge. The "lights" of G0d and of Soul are lights that have application under all circumstances and for all healing. Life and healing are optimized by incorporating these crucial concepts. Absence of these lights in healthcare will cause us to seek substitute lights which may seem bright, but which will often leave us in the wrong place including receiving unnecessary and inappropriate surgery, disability, and even death.

Understanding this concept might be helped with an analogy using lights with which we are all familiar. Everyone is thankful for streetlights that help us see and be safe while walking and driving at night. But few if any of us are excited when we see streetlights despite their great safety value for us. The lights of fireworks which are often used for celebration, yet have no functional value, arouse great excitement.

The eternal lights of G0d and Soul, although lifesaving, like the streetlights, are often ignored and not recognized. The lights of fireworks are purely for show without any intrinsic value, yet crowds come from far and near to witness them. Marketing in healthcare, business, law, etc. often tends to exaggerate the value of a service or product by creating fireworks-like excitement. This marketing "fireworks" intentionally or not is often a distraction from truth which goes hand in hand with the lights of G0d and Soul.

3

That Tied Up Feeling

Happiness and contentment are not beyond reach. But some of us are unhappy with our weight. Some of us don't like the way we look. Some of us don't like the way we feel. Perhaps you've read diet books, magazines, and articles, followed diets, and enrolled in diet companies. You've changed the way you eat over and over. You've even received prepared meals in the mail. You've taken diet pills. You've followed exercise recommendations. Perhaps you've undergone weight reduction surgery. Ultimately, you're no better than when you started. You might even be worse off. You're not happy with yourself or the way things are. Do you feel like you're all tied up and you and your life are stuck?

Life is, by nature, a "tied up" situation. Tied and diet have the same four letters. Rearrange the letters in "d-i-e-t," and you have "t-i-e-d." What does it mean to be "tied up?" It means to be unnecessarily constrained and restricted. We all experienced birth, a process none of us had any say in and which requires three partners: Mom, Dad, and G0d. Mom and Dad provide the physical genetics for the body, and G0d provides a tiny piece of Himself to inhabit your body. This piece provided by G0d is your Divine essence and is the real you known as the Soul.

The Soul is restricted by and confined to your body throughout this lifetime, and in this way, your body acts as a prison to the Soul. People are always looking for ways to escape their "tied-upness." Surfing all day, boating, playing music, doing art, yoga, exercise, prayer, and other activities are pursued as healthy ways to transcend our bodily prisons and achieve an "out-of-body" experience, a freeing of the real you, the Soul.

The body is but the first layer of restriction for the Soul. Additional restrictions come from all our layers of connections. A healthy body is less restrictive than a body challenged by congenital or acquired disease, trauma, or disability. Then there is the restrictive need some have for orthotics or prosthetics. From the Soul's perspective, continuing outward in restrictive concentric layers there is your body with its skin, hair, and nails, makeup, clothes, car, and home. Restricting relationships include spouse, children, parents, siblings, cousins, uncles and aunts, friends, and community.

Our choice of work and work relationships are also significant restrictions. Many restricting interactions occur while driving your car. Your cell phone with phone, text, email, Facebook, Twitter, LinkedIn, Instagram, and many apps plays a huge role today in restricting people, as do all of our technologies, machines, and possessions. Some or all of these technologies may, at times, seem liberating, and in fact many have the stated purpose and are in fact vehicles for allowing communication and connection. However, at all times they restrict the Soul's power of expression through thought, speech, and action in time and place.

The ordinary person is tied up from birth till death and few can extricate themselves from an identity that they never chose for themselves. You didn't choose to be born. You didn't choose your body. You didn't choose your parents, family, relatives, or community. You didn't choose the time or location of your arrival on the scene. You learned from your parents, relatives, teachers, friends and their families, tv, movies, media, and the surrounding prevailing culture. You lived up to a variety of expectations. You went to school. You sought a job and a career. You sought a spouse, children, and a home. You thought and did what you were molded to do.

And every choice and pathway tied you up more and more. In this respect, your path was the same as everyone else's. It was what you were expected to do and what everyone else did. But who are you really? What is your identity?

Our tied-up life with so many restrictions can be overwhelming. Many of our encumbrances are imposed on us from sources outside of ourselves and are unavoidable. Yet, many of our limitations are self-imposed and are a direct result of our life choices and decisions. It is imperative that we learn the importance of making wise choices and gain the skill to do so early in life to avoid a life filled with anxiety and pain. A regular thorough evaluation and stock-taking of one's life is important to help you be all you can be by minimizing externally and internally directed restrictions.

Have you been living as the real you? Have you been living the life you really would have wanted to live, or do you feel like a programmed robot? Do you feel like you have a say in directing your life or do you feel like life merely happens to you? Have you been truly living or merely existing? Who has been making your decisions for you? Has it been others who have molded your expectations and desires? Have you given over your Soul Power to others or perhaps to parts of your own body including your brain, heart, or the rest of your body? How do you decide what to think, say, and do?

From a young age, we get exposed to things that we can choose to allow into our lives or to keep out. Cigarettes, alcohol, and drugs are some of these. We know that these things are harmful to us, and therefore the smartest choice is to "Just say no." But vast numbers of people partake of these things. When they get smart and decide to stop, too often they can't. They have let themselves get tied up in something that seems more powerful than them. Could it be that a rolled piece of paper with tobacco inside, or a bottle of alcohol, or a pill or other form of drug is more powerful than a human being? It appears so. How is this possible?

Eating is different from smoking, drinking alcohol, and using drugs. Eating is essential for life, whereas the others are not. Expressions used to describe overeating or addictive eating are "eating like a pig" and "eating like an animal." These phrases really mean that the person has no self-control and can refer to the choice of food as well as the amount of food. There is a problem with these descriptions though. Pigs and animals have limited food choices, and they stop eating when their physical hunger has been satisfied. Pigs and animals don't eat like pigs and animals. Only human beings "eat like pigs and animals."

In recent times, and for the first time in recorded history, obesity has become a worldwide epidemic for children and adults of all ages. One would think that since we are more intellectually, scientifically, and technologically advanced than previous generations, we would not have this problem. People who are overweight or obese are often not happy with their weight, appearance, life, marriage, divorce, parents, children, job, or any collection of issues that all of us deal with at one time or another.

There are innumerable diet books, magazines, blogs, diets, plans, companies, apps, supplements and pills, meals, surgeries, and more to subscribe to. Many millions of people are fighting obesity worldwide and there are many so-called solutions. Nonetheless, studies and research suggest that the very profitable business of weight loss is one big scam and is all about taking advantage of troubled people purely for profit. The diet and weight loss industry is an eighty billion dollar business in America alone and that dollar figure has historically been on a steady rise. This figure does not include the medical cost for treatment of all the diseases that result from and are associated with obesity.

"Just say no" applies equally well to cigarettes, alcohol, drugs, and food. It's all about having self-control. Can all the diet books, plans, and companies sell you self-control? Where does self-control come from? Is it learned, genetic, or developed? Does it exist in the body, the heart, the brain, or the Soul? How does all of this really work? Is there something missing with all the diet business stuff? What about addiction and recovery? Is there a better way? The problems of obesity and addiction are the focus of the weight loss and addiction recovery industries. As we explore these and other devastating problems along with the industries associated with them, we will consider alternative solutions to many of humanity's dilemmas.

More:

When I was a young boy and was invited to parties or was in any social or school setting, I felt different from everyone else and they let me know I was different. I knew I was quiet, and they called me shy. A group of girls in my class sent me a regular dose of cards with the letters S.M.I.L.E. and some kind of a note encouraging me to smile. I didn't like to speak, and I guess that I adopted my mother's habit of wearing a serious face.

When food, snacks, or candy were available I prided myself on having the discipline to refuse them. When the other kids began partaking in cigarettes, alcohol, and drugs, this behavior always seemed foolish to me and I simply ignored them and focused on my own healthy interests. Therefore, self-control with my mouth and in life generally was easy and natural for me.

I am sure that this self-control and discipline at an early age was somehow the result of my sensitivity to my mother's Holocaust experience and her emotional pain. I was always smart and sometimes wise for my age and wanted to be the best and healthiest I could be for my own betterment. I also tried to be at my best behavior to please my mother and not cause her any more pain than she'd already experienced. By doing so, I hoped to somehow wage battle against, conquer, and correct the evil that had been done to my mother, her family, and the six million Jews murdered in the Holocaust including one and one-half million children. Self-control and discipline in behavior, relationships, academia, music, and sports gave me a sense of strength, courage, and power that I would need to combat evil and pain.

4

We Need A New Paradigm

For generations, discipline was taught and passed down in families from parents to children and culturally from one generation to the next. The key discipline was always respecting and honoring parents and elders. Children knew their parents and elders were older and wiser and, therefore, closer to G0d. Honor and respect for parents and elders also meant honor and respect for G0d. But this relationship between the young and their elders and G0d has changed in the last two generations.

Immigrants to America, from a variety of countries, did not speak English and generally did not have college degrees. Their children did learn to speak English and went to college. Perhaps for the first time in history, the parents assumed that their English-speaking college-educated children knew more than them, and their children knew they knew more than their parents. Suddenly the age-old respect for parents and the elderly disappeared. Also thrown into the waste bin of history was the long-valued respect for G0d.

Simultaneous with the lack of respect for parents, the elderly, and G0d came the lack of self- respect. Instead of self-respect, self-worship with a focus on "me," pursuing careers for monetary success, and the "shark" mentality all came into vogue. Self-respect, self-discipline, self-control, and the ability to "just say no" took a back seat to seeking bodily pleasure. Human beings transformed from Soul beings to bodily pleasure seekers. Pleasure based on bodily physical feelings and on physical possessions superseded human qualities and values which had been developed and held by our parents and for generations before us. The way of life that was considered extremely important for human health and survival of the family, communities, culture, morality, and civilization, was abandoned.

People suddenly expected a quick answer and a quick fix for everything. They could eat anything and violate age-old mores. Smoking, drinking, drugs, tattoos, piercings, relationships and sexual adventure in unchartered territory, and any physical bodily pleasure became acceptable and desirable. But with lack of discipline and respect for self, others, and G0d come multiple disease epidemics, depression, emptiness, helplessness, hopelessness, and loneliness. Although some quick fixes work, there are no quick fixes for many of the problems we have created. The big problem today is not the environment or the diseases we have created. It is the inability of human beings to find our way back to discipline, respect, acts of lovingkindness, and G0d. We have abandoned our G0d-given potential to realize our identities as Divine Souls.

We have allowed the human being to be reduced to just what we can see with our eyes-a body with a shape and size. People are under the misconception that we are merely a body with physical needs. But we are so much more than that. Yes, we have a body that is made up of a collection of miraculous living machines that ordinarily function in a finely tuned and inter-coordinated manner. The brain is a physical organ which is the seat of our intellect. It is the powerful and intricate divinely designed computer that oversees our bodily functions and actions. The heart is a physical organ that must miraculously work nonstop 24-7-365 throughout our entire life to sustain our life and is the seat of our emotions. The other organ systems are responsible for our other bodily functions.

We know our body must take in food and drink to survive. But why and how has obesity become such a huge problem? Clearly, we have lost self-discipline and self-control. The battle we face with obesity is not with food. Similarly, the struggle we face with cigarette smoking, alcoholism, drug addiction, and other similar problems is not with cigarettes, alcohol, or drugs. The battle is one with ourselves. It is an internal battle. Let's examine the battlefield.

The current assumption by the diet industry is that all hunger is physical hunger. You are your body. Your body is hungry. So, you eat. If you are merely a body, then you are only physical matter. But the essential "you" is nonphysical. We are Soul entities that temporarily reside in our bodies. Many people are unaware that they are a Soul. Some people think they have a Soul. But you don't have a Soul. You are the Soul.

The Soul resides in your body which is no more you than your car or your home or a spacesuit you might wear would be considered you. The deception that we are our body occurs because unlike our cars, homes, and spacesuits which we can freely enter and exit, we are "locked in" to our bodies for a prolonged period of time amounting to our entire lifetime. This approach to the Soul and body is just the beginning in the development of a different way of understanding who we are as human beings, how we work as Soul and body, and how we interact with the world around us.

The Soul has certain functions similar to the body. The Soul feeds, it grows, and it gives off waste. When we live as the Soul and know how to feed our Soul, we can find a healthy balance of Soul and body. But what happens when the Soul is hungry, yet we are only aware of our body. We interpret this Soul hunger as bodily hunger and feed our bodies. But Soul hunger is never satisfied with physical food. So, we keep eating and never stop. The result is worldwide obesity epidemics in adults and children. We have relinquished our true identity as our G0dly selves for an identity as our physical bodies.

If you see yourself as merely your body, then you can readily conclude that you are what you eat because the molecules of what you eat become incorporated into your body, which you consider to be yourself. If you are cognizant of your existence as the Soul and know how to feed your Soul, then you will not be on an endless path of eating physical food to satisfy your Soul hunger. But if you identify as your body and eat to satisfy both physical and Soul hunger, then you have created a never-ending relationship with food. You have allowed yourself to become and be defined by your overweight or obese body and the food you eat.

Like a child that has only physical needs and looks to its parents to satisfy those needs, the overweight, obese person has relinquished their ability to control themselves. Like an infant who cannot meet its own needs and must rely on its parents, the overweight obese person looks to diets, diet books, diet fads, diet plans, diet companies, diet pills, and weight loss surgery for help. Yet, we know that none of these heavily marketed solutions are statistically successful in the long run.

The problem of abdication of self-control is not unique to people struggling with their weight, their self-image, and their seeming control by the food they eat. A similar problem exists also for people troubled by mental health issues, pain, cigarette addiction, coffee addiction, alcohol addiction, drug addiction, and addictions of all types. Of course, exceptions exist, and whereas lack of self-control may be a sign of weakness for some, for others it is a lack of education.

The collective businesses of mental health, pain evaluation and treatment, and cigarette, alcohol, and drug sales and addiction management probably total in the hundreds of billions to trillions of dollars. The answer to solving all of these problems generally, of course with some rare exceptions, is self-control. In the past, self-control and the ability to master oneself was a source of happiness and pleasure.

Today, people are deceived into thinking that meaning and happiness come from things of the physical world that we all can see-things outside of our Soul selves. People have come to think that to be happy you must have a more beautiful or more muscular body, even if it results from taking drugs or undergoing plastic surgery, expensive clothes, cars, and homes, high-paying professional jobs with their accompanying titles, a larger bank book, etc. It has become all about "ME," "I want," and "I need."

The children brought into the world today are being educated to believe the nonsense and lies that their parents have adopted. Since parents have come to believe that material possessions are the source of happiness, they give their children everything they want including every new toy, game, technology, and possession. Discipline and self-control are not values understood or held by parents generally, so they do not teach these important concepts to their children. Parents are aided in their education of children that the search for happiness depends on acquiring material positions by the way fancy and expensive clothes, cars, homes, etc. are marketed. To my knowledge, self-control is not marketed.

Instead of understanding the great value of teaching a child self-restraint, discipline, and self-control, parents generally feel they would be depriving their child of happiness and love if they did so. But just the reverse is true. By giving a child lessons in these values, the child will more readily learn self-esteem and lovingkindness. Self-esteem allows contentment with oneself and with life generally regardless of possessions. Happiness then becomes a mental attitude rather than a result of having stuff.

The truthful solutions to so many mind-boggling and costly problems plaguing humanity have been elusive. These problems include obesity, mental health, pain evaluation and treatment, cigarette, alcohol, drug, and food addiction, corporate and organizational wellness, sedentary disease, achieving and maintaining physical fitness, Alzheimer's Disease and senile dementia of aging, and the explosion in the number of surgeries based on MRI results. They demand a different approach with a different paradigm from the currently acclaimed experts, companies, and products. The solution process requires the ability to see the beauty of the entire vast forest for the trees.

The experts of today are typically educated and trained in a very tunnel-vision way and, as a result of this process, often do not see the forest. They do not even see the trees. Many have been whittled down in their own lives in the course of their education and training and have lost the potential for total humanity they once possessed as children.

The experts trained as medical professionals, both in allopathic traditional physical medicine and in complementary alternative medicine, and other healthcare professionals and business professionals, are generally so tunnel-vision oriented that at best they see pieces of sawdust rather than the trees or the forest. Rarely, they may see small carved-out pieces of a tree the size of toothpicks. But for these professionals to see an entire tree or collection of trees, let alone the broader vast beautiful forest is rare. Often these professionals and experts have the same or similar problems that they purport to know how to treat. They have lost touch with the human issues causing so many problems. Instead of creating effective ways to solve and prevent problems, they resort to turning everyone's problems into the problem they are trained to treat.

The experts and us have a big perspective problem. We both are deceived into thinking that "you are what you see" and "seeing is believing." On the contrary, however, you are not what you see. Don't let what you see deceive you. Your body that you see is the wrapper-the container-the vessel-the conduit-for the real you. Your real self-your essence-your true identity-is the Soul that your body houses. You don't have a Soul. You are the Soul. And you as the Soul have a body. The Soul is hidden and cannot be seen. It is the G0d-given fruit contained by the body. The body is merely the peel. Yet, in this physical world we temporarily inhabit, the Soul cannot accomplish anything without using the body. The Soul must actualize its purpose and mission by utilizing the body. The key is to understand who we are as Soul identities and how we as Soul entities can optimally, meaningfully, efficiently, wisely, and happily utilize our G0d-given and genetically programmed bodies to accomplish our earthly mission. To do so we must know our purpose in our limited time visiting earth?

More:

In my early years my father taught me the story of a man wielding an axe to chop a tree in the woods. A passerby watched the man chopping and saw that he wasn't making much progress. He suggested that he stop chopping to sharpen his axe. The man replied that he didn't have time.

So many of us become comfortable in our current station in life that we accept our "baggage" with our "luggage." We become used to the stuff we should eject or fix rather than taking the time to better ourselves. A time out to rethink, learn, strengthen, and fortify ourselves so that we can return to our mission with renewed strength and a healthier outlook is always worthwhile.

This lesson is always relevant, and I consider it especially so when dealing with our own pain and problems. I also believe this story is relevant for science, medicine, and the doctors and experts who have time-honored ways of understanding and doing things. A revolution and upheaval in our understanding and ways of doing things, if for the better, should always be welcome.

A related story of prioritization in life involves a professor who presents to his class with a large glass jar. He fills it with large stones and askes the class if it's full. When they say yes, he adds many pebbles until the jar will not accommodate any more, and again asks them if it's full. When they say yes, he fills the jar with sand and once again asks them if it's full. They are hesitant to respond. When they say yes, he fills the jar with beer. He then explains to them that filling the jar is a lesson about priorities in life.

In life we are limited in time and space. If the beer, sand, or pebbles preceded the larger stones, there would not have been room for all of the stones or possibly any of them. A key lesson in life is to devote time and space to our important priorities first and only then pursue lesser priorities. Prioritizing our thought, speech, and action is crucial for success in life. Then the students asked why beer was used in the lesson and the professor responded that naturally, it's always a good time for a beer.

Success in seeing the forest for the trees and in prioritizing one's life in time and space would be a monumental accomplishment for anyone. The beer accompanying this successful approach to life is symbolic of happiness, joy, and thankfulness for the ability to lead a meaningful and purposeful life.

5

The New Paradigm
(Old Paradigm Revisited)

We have addressed the need to see ourselves as a nonphysical Soul, a minuscule piece of G0d, housed in a physical body. But how do we do this? What are the tools at our disposal? A simple analogy exists. We as nonphysical Soul entities can choose to use different parts of our bodies to actualize a given process. This is similar to being in your home with all kinds of technological devices at your disposal. We can choose to use or not use a given device. Similarly, we can choose to turn a device on or off. We can decide how to use a device, when to turn it on, how we interact with it, how we let it affect us, how long we use it, and when to turn it off.

Consider your cell phone, pad, laptop, or computer. You can control these devices, and if you desire, you can always gain more skills to do so. You have the same ability to learn, be trained, and train yourself to control your brain, and you are always capable of increasing your skillset. You can turn your brain function on or off. You can use it to scan old memory files or record new ones. You can use it to analyze information and draw con-clusions. All the modern technological devices at home are at our disposal to use as we desire. They do not function independently. Similarly, our bodily organ systems require monitoring by our Soul essence for optimal function to accomplish our goals and mission.

Those people who don't realize or acknowledge their Soul essence may live purely in the physical realm. Instead of empowering the Soul in the driver's seat of life, they give over control of bodily function to their bodily organs themselves. They allow their brain to control and determine their thoughts and intellect. They empower their heart as the seat of their emotions to manage their feelings. They empower their stomach to dictate eating habits. They empower the doctors and the healthcare system with their health. They empower gyms, fitness equipment manufacturers, and personal trainers with their fitness and exercise programs. The Soul can wisely dictate how all these tools are used or it can blindly go along for the ride.

This approach can be understood with the analogy of the horse and buggy. The buggy has a carriage in which rides the passenger who has commissioned the horse and buggy to journey from one place to another. This passenger determines where the buggy will go. The driver of the buggy is required to lead the horse in the right direction and control his pace. He is only driving because it is his job and he will be paid. He is not invested in the trip or where they are going other than he is required to provide a pleasant journey, and he might treat himself to food and drink at the destination. The horse does not have a choice whether to participate and ordinarily is treated with food and water at the destination.

Imagine that after the passenger gets in the carriage, he does not in-struct the driver where he wants to go. He instead lets the driver and horse determine what to do and where to go, and he assumes he's going to get to his desired destination. Perhaps he doesn't even have a destination in mind. In this model the passenger represents our Soul which is a temporary passenger in our body, the driver represents our brain and intellect, the horse represents our heart and emotions, and the carriage represents the rest of our body in which is found the Soul.

Letting the driver and horse control the journey will rarely if ever get the passenger to the desired destination. Although this conclusion is evident regarding the horse and buggy, and no one would accept to be a passenger and leave the unchartered journey to the whim of the driver and horse, this is how many people lead their lives. They are ignorant of or abdicate their role as Soul represented by the passenger in the carriage. Instead of taking commanding control of the body and bodily organs represented by the driver, horse, and carriage, they let the driver, horse, and carriage, representing the brain, heart, and other bodily organs, control them. Just as the driver and horse may crave food or drink, many people let their physical cravings control them rather than empowering the Soul.

The Soul has the power to exert control over the brain, intellect, and thought, the heart, emotions, and feelings, the nose and smell, the eyes and sight, the ears and hearing, the mouth, speech, and eating, and the arms and legs and a large variety of activities. The Soul can also prevent and control any cravings. Choosing to live and actualize one's life as the Soul gives each and every one of us the ability or Soul Power to exert willpower, self-control, and discipline over the bodily organs and their functions. Negating the existence of Soul also negates the Soul Power with which we are all endowed. G0d blesses us with this power so that we can be of use to G0d as a helpmate. G0d wants us each to find our Soul Identity and Soul Power to serve G0d's purpose in creating us.

More:

When G0d made the world, it is written that He said, "Let us make man." Who could the "us" possibly have been if G0d was the only One in existence? One possibility is that He was speaking to the angels. An explanation that resonates with me more is that He was speaking to the Souls of humanity which were, of course, a part of Himself. The profound aspect of G0d's statement is that G0d would place the Divine Souls in human bodies, and then the Souls would be responsible throughout life to "make man." They would have to validate their existence in this physical world as human beings by showing what they were truly made of. This would be a lifelong mission of bringing G0dliness into their physical lives and revealing the G0dliness in the physical world. This is an obligation, perhaps even a covenant, between G0d and humankind.

To accomplish this mission, we must see ourselves as more than just "mind and body." Some give token credence to soul and equate soul, mind, and body. But we all can aspire to know ourselves as the higher Soul entities we are. Once we accept this paradigm for ourselves, we can learn to rule over our intellect and emotions rather than being controlled by them. Balance is achieved by establishing a Soul relationship with G0d and using the mind, heart, and body in the service of G0d.

6

The Soul-Body Relationship

Our paradigm has shifted from identifying as a body seeking physical pleasure and happiness from material things to a nonphysical Soul cloaked in a body. The body is a delicately arranged collection of integrated living technological machines for the Soul to use to actualize its purpose. The Soul has a continual relationship with the body for the duration of one's life, and each body part has immeasurable value to each one of us. Yet, many people take their body parts and organs for granted. Most of us know more about our possessions such as eyeglasses, watch, clothes, cellphone, laptop, car, etc. than we know about our own body parts. It is certainly important to know how things work. What could be more important than understanding the Soul and body relationship and how the Soul uses our body parts to accomplish its mission?

The brain is a physical body part. Its functions are collectively known as the mind or intellect. It is the seat of memory, thought, analysis, reasoning, deliberation, understanding, decision-making, dreaming, and more. The Soul uses the brain for these processes. Lack of understanding of the relationship between the Soul and brain can lead to one's brain leading the Soul. You can empower your brain to supplant the Soul and let it run your life. This way of living is analogous to allowing the driver of the horse and buggy to take you wherever he wants to go rather than you as the paying passenger determining your destination. To empower you as Soul to take command of your brain, it helps to know how this relationship works and how the brain functions in the service of the Soul.

The Soul must exhibit desire, intention, drive, willpower, strength, and courage to pursue its mission and purpose. These qualities enable the Soul to utilize and master control of the brain and the entire body. The life of the Soul is actualized by using its body to interact with the world through three vehicles-thought, speech, and action. Everything we humans are about is some combination of these three activities. Thought, speech, and action are best accomplished when they are managed by the Soul, beginning first with the brain, the bodily organ of thought and intellect. When the Soul abdicates its power to the body and allows bodily organs and bodily desires to overtake control of the brain and control of thought, speech, and action, that's when problems arise.

The Soul has the capacity to use the brain to formulate and program the rest of the body for living. The Soul can empower the brain to help it think. Any use of the brain activates the process of thought. Three steps are followed to fully actualize the process of our Soul using our brain to create thought, speech, and action. The first step requires formulation of an idea.

Regardless of what you want to think, say, or do, you must first draw an idea down into your brain from the well of potential infinite ideas. This idea involves expression of a desire to think about something, to speak about something, or to perform some bodily action. The Soul has the power to grasp this idea and act on it or to shut it down immediately. Should the Soul be pleased with the idea, then a second step consisting of understanding how to actualize the idea must occur. Whether the desired thought, speech, or action is familiar or new, reading, learning, observing, and practicing it will give the Soul feedback as to whether it is pleased with its choice.

The third step involves the Soul's experience of pleasure or displeasure accompanying the thought, speech, or action. The Soul's reaction will determine whether it will pursue this pathway again or not. All thought, speech, and action evolve via this sequential process of idea formation, understanding and actualization, and resultant biofeedback. The Soul has the power to then embrace the thought, speech, or action and generate a green go-ahead light resulting in a positive feedback loop promoting the behavior. Alternatively, the Soul can generate a red stoplight resulting in a negative feedback loop with discontinuation of the behavior.

The Soul also has the ability to empower the heart and emotions. Emotions consist of two extremes and a wide variety of intermediates which are some blend of the two. On one extreme is a desire to bond, unite, or connect with someone, something, or a thought process, and this emotion or feeling is known as love. On the opposite extreme is a desire to flee, escape, disconnect, or run from someone, something, or a thought process, and this emotion or feeling is known as fear or pain. It is said that emotions and feelings originate in the heart and perhaps this is so, but ultimately, they become thoughts and are processed by the brain.

Under the best of circumstances, you are the Soul and are in command of your G0d-given tools including your brain and intellect, and your heart and emotions. In this capacity you can choose to use your intellect to rule over your feelings or alternatively you can empower your emotions to rule over your intellect. The intellect can evaluate and temper emotions, which are short term reactions to life occurrences. The emotions do not have this same ability to assess the intellect. The intellect is, therefore, the higher seat of function, and it follows that the wise approach in life is for the Soul to utilize the intellect to rule over the emotions.

Throughout our lives, we can develop our intellect and our emotions and our capacity to manage their relationship. The Soul's ability to govern it's intellectual and emotional prowess will determine its success in its relations with others, things, thought processes, and life generally. If the Soul abandons its role and gives full power to intellect or emotions, then life can be haphazard.

Let's see how the relationship between Soul, intellect, and emotions works concerning eating. The Soul can use the intellect to evaluate different eating possibilities and make healthy choices. These healthy choices might include limiting or avoiding meat, carbohydrates, sugar, fat, soda, and processed foods, eating primarily fruits and vegetables, not food shopping when hungry, eating and chewing slowly, serving oneself small portions, and only eating when hungry and not because it is a given time or food is available.

The emotions won't necessarily go along with this wise collection of choices and might naturally prefer meat, sugars and sweets, carbohydrates and fats, sodas and processed foods, and eating fast and to excess. The Soul has the power to use the intellect to decide on the best path for good health, wellness, and happiness and then must guide the intellect to overrule the emotions. When this is practiced repetitively over time, the emotions can be trained to line up in support of the intellect, and the process of eating becomes a collection of healthy habits.

If the Soul doesn't take charge but instead abdicates its power to the intellect and the emotions, havoc can result in uncontrolled weight gain and obesity and a variety of subsequent health problems. These include heart disease, hypertension, diabetes, muscle and joint pain and arthritis, inflammation, and more. The intellect can be influenced by cultural, societal, and food business marketing techniques. These commonly promote eating three meals a day, the importance of a large breakfast, the best times to eat, how much to eat and drink of various foods, food types, and drinks, how much water to drink, and more. The Soul can use the brain to evaluate these choices and make its own decisions or it can merely empower the intellect to follow these choices. If the Soul and intellect are left out of the process and eating is an emotional process, then the mouth will follow the eyes and eating will more than likely be anything but healthy.

We have all been brought up with the cultural norms to eat three meals a day, and that breakfast is the most important meal of the day. Many people follow these tenets without ever questioning them. With a little thought and experimentation, eating sparsely and healthfully and only when hungry, whenever that may be, regardless of the time, may be a better, wiser, and healthier plan than sticking to breakfast, lunch, and dinner at fixed times.

If dinner or a late meal is eaten and is not followed by vigorous activity, that digested meal is still available in the morning to invigorate the first part of the day. The morning is the best part of the day to be motivated and energized to get a lot accomplished. If a large breakfast is eaten then the gut will pool blood from the rest of the body, including the brain, to allow for digestion, and you will become sluggish and sleepy. This behavior will counter any desire to make the morning meaningful. But in line with so many commercials we have heard over the years, it will sell eggs, milk, orange juice, bread, butter, margarine, cereal, pancake mix, and more. A better and healthier choice might be to limit any food intake in the morning until you have first met your morning goals and then when hungry eat a modest healthy meal.

It all comes back to discipline and training. We each must know our identity as a Divine Soul temporarily riding in the body with our intellect and emotions and all of our bodily functions at our disposal. The highest form of existence to optimize our health, wellness, and happiness is for us as Soul entities to utilize our intellect to evaluate and process our worldly existence including our emotions. Allowing our emotions to control us without oversight by Soul and intellect is a lower form of existence preventing us from rising to our true potential. Regardless of our past, we always have the potential with each new moment to utilize our greater understanding to create a new life of discipline and sound healthy choices.

More:

Eating is essential for life. It is like breathing air. It is similar to putting gas in the gas tank and without which the car won't go. Yet the necessity to eat to live, survive, and thrive can be turned into something totally different. The same action of eating that we cannot live without and which can be done responsibly, healthfully, and efficiently can be turned into a selfish time to please the body. We learn this mode of pleasing the body with food when Mom makes big tasty meals, especially at holidays like Thanksgiving. Many of us learn to gorge ourselves on all kinds of unhealthy foods that taste good and on unhealthy amounts of these foods.

Once we have a physically pleasurable experience, it becomes a challenge to relegate that kind of experience to only specific set times in the year. Maintaining discipline and knowing how to "just say no" is a very valuable skill. Our Moms do not mean to mess up our lives by overfeeding us with delectable delicacies at certain times. But it can be just one exposure to a holiday meal that triggers a lifelong lack of discipline and lack of control of the mouth. It is typical of physical pleasures of all types that there is no natural ceiling or endpoint to satisfaction. The mantra often becomes, "the more the merrier." One who has one wants two. Who has two wants four. And who has four wants eight, etc. The easiest and safest way to prevent this mistake is at the very beginning to "just say no" and be sure that once one chooses to partake in any path or pleasure one follows the wiser mantra of "everything in moderation."

7

The Mouth

The organs of the head governing connection with the outside world are our two eyes, two ears, two nostrils, and one mouth. One explanation for the duality of eyes, ears, and nostrils is that one eye is to see good and one is to see bad, one ear is to hear good and one is to hear bad, and one nostril is to smell good and one is to smell bad. Theoretically this concept would allow one to easily separate good from bad and focus on the good. But there is only one mouth. Everything that we say and eat, both good and bad, has to pass through this one portal. The mouth has no obvious ready mechanism to separate good from bad.

The eyes, ears, and nose are open in their natural resting state, allowing us to be sensitive to sensory stimuli. Yet when the stimuli are not healthy, we have mechanisms to avoid them. The eyes can easily close or be covered by a hand, the ears can be easily plugged with the earlobes or with a finger or by covering them with your hands, and the nostrils can be squeezed shut or covered by a hand. The anatomic machinery of the mouth is relatively complex and unlike the other organs of the head is closed in its natural resting state.

The anatomy of the mouth seems to be constructed to promote its closure, almost as if it were a fortress that needs to be protected from ingress or egress. Energy must be exerted to open the mouth. It is a monster machine with several barrier walls whose function seems more to prevent than to promote passage through it. The tongue and the palate are anatomically important for eating and speech. The upper and lower rows of teeth and the upper and lower lips act as impassable walls when closed. They can be reinforced inside by plugging with the tongue and outside by a hand.

The functions of the mouth are primarily two-fold: eating and speech. Eating is essential for the survival of the body. Speech is essential for communicating with others. Both eating and speaking are essential for thriving in our complex world. The major problem with obesity is an inability to limit the passage of food into the mouth. This is a lack of self-discipline to control the mouth. The mouth is a "two-way street" so that if one lacks control of the inflow of food, more than likely, there will be a concomitant lack of control of outflow of speech.

Although both speech and food are vital for life, there are speech and food that are supportive of healthy living and there are those that are harmful and even deadly. It is said that speaking about someone who is not present, known as gossip, causes harm to the speaker, the listener, and the one spoken about. Words must be carefully thought out, chosen, focused, and delivered to have the desired effect. Similarly, food put into one's mouth should be chosen to be of a particular type, quality, and quantity. The more health oriented these choices are, the healthier will be the outcome.

Self-constraint and self-discipline with one's mouth are worthy practices. Speech and food are best in limited quantity and carefully chosen quality. Just because something is permissible to be said or eaten, that is precisely the perfect time to practice self-restraint and keep the mouth closed. That time is always. This self-restraint especially applies to speaking toxic words and eating unhealthy food.

Keeping the mouth closed is perhaps the best practice for adults and children to gain self-control, self-mastery, self-esteem, health, wellness, and happiness. It is no wonder that much addiction of all types involves a lack of self-control with one's mouth. In addiction, the mouth transforms from a strong barrier to an uncontrolled thoroughfare. Food, speech, cigarettes, alcohol, and drugs require abstention or moderation by the ability to "just say no." This self-control is accomplished by the Soul, brain and intellect, heart and emotions, and mouth and by keeping the mouth blockaded shut in its resting state.

Teaching children self-control and self-discipline regarding use of the mouth for speech and eating would go a long way to preventing addiction problems and relationship problems. Rather than living to eat, speak, and engage in oral habits abundantly, the mouth would be put to better use by eating, speaking, and doing everything it engages in with discipline and moderation to create an abundant life.

More:

Have you heard the joke about the man who wanted to become a monk? He went to the monastery and was told by the abbot, or head monk, that he must take a vow of silence and could only say two words every three years. He agreed. After the first three years, the abbot came to him and asked him what his first two words were. "Food cold!" he replied. The abbot then made sure the meals were not cold. After three more years the abbot came to him and asked him for his two words. "No rice!" was his reply. The abbot then provided food substitutes for rice. After another three years the abbot approached him for his next two words. "Fish dry!" he responded, and the abbot made sure the fish was moist. Three more years went by and the abbot asked him for his two words. "I quit!" he exclaimed. The abbot declared, "Well, I'm not surprised. You've done nothing but complain since you got here."

The life of a monk is all about mastering self-control. This humorous story conveys the ability to speak few words and keep the mouth closed. It is consistent with the notion that self-control may be most readily acquired when one practices minimal use of the mouth.

8

No, You're Not Crazy

Have you ever felt disjointed as if you are two different people with different conflicting drives and motivations? Well, in effect, you are. We each are one person with two different Souls and two different Soul natures residing in our singular body. One Soul is the one we have been discussing that is an infinitesimal piece of G0d endowed to us by G0d Himself to live our purpose in the service of G0d. This Soul is selfless and has the sole mission to serve G0d. This Soul is known as the G0dly or Divine Soul. The second Soul is intrinsic to the body. Just as every creation has its own Soul and animals have animal Souls, since our body is of an animal nature, this second Soul can be called the animal Soul. This Soul is selfish and lives for the pleasure of the body.

The Divine Soul and the animal Soul both reside in the same body, yet their natural missions clash. The Divine Soul has the sole purpose and drive to use the body selflessly in the service of G0d. The Animal Soul is about using the body selfishly in the service of the pleasure of the body. The Divine Soul desires for you to be the best, kindest, most helpful human being you can be for G0d, yourself, your family, your community, and the world. The animal Soul is all about "I" and "me" and feeling physically content without regard for your health and welfare, and without concern for G0d or anyone else. All that matters is the sense of pleasure experienced by the body, and the animal Soul will seek to use the body to attain that sense of pleasure in any way possible.

The prime seat of function of the Divine Soul is in the brain and the intellect. The Divine Soul uses the brain and intellect to be humble, modest, thoughtful, careful, meditative, pensive, deliberate, and kind in its use of the body to actualize its purpose. In contrast, the prime seat of function of the animal Soul is the heart and the emotions. The Animal Soul uses the heart and emotions to be selfish, careless, impulsive, unrestrained, undisciplined, and insatiable in its use of the body. The Divine Soul does not live for physical food and instead lives for the nourishment of the Soul. The animal Soul has a natural desire to please the body with physical food.

The Divine Soul is not interested in the body beyond satisfying the need to keep the body healthy for healthy living and using the body for good works. The animal Soul, however, is a different story. It thrives on physical pleasures such as food and eating. The animal Soul is not interested in disciplined eating such as limiting oneself to healthy food, small portions, or only eating when hungry. The animal Soul's motto is, "If it feels good to me, nothing else matters! I'm doing it!" This desire for any and all physical pleasures, including but not limited to food, speech, cigarettes, alcohol, and drugs, knows no bounds.

Now you must all be most thankful to know that we are all "schizophrenic" by nature with split personalities. With two opposing personalities competing for use of our singular body and its organs and component parts to satisfy their distinct and different life's missions, how is anyone to lead a productive life? It is problematic enough to have two separate people such as husband and wife or two business partners who are supposed to get along have their relationship turn into a battle. Such a struggle can wreak havoc on the relationship.

What are we to do when this type of battle is being waged within us between our Divine and animal Souls? As our basest nature, some of us humans prefer to live like animals driven by the animal Soul totally ignoring the Divine Soul. Others of us live a balance of both contrasting motivations. Fewer of us live primarily as the Divine Soul.

One of these pathways is easy and takes no work. It is the "natural" way. The opposite path requires understanding, self-discipline, and a lot of work. The natural route is the path of least resistance and is about just doing what feels good to the body. This is the level of the mentality of the infant that only lives for the satisfaction of its bodily needs and pleasure. This is the lower level of functioning of the human being as the animal Soul. Then there is the higher level of functioning as the Divine Soul. The physical pleasure of the body is no longer the driving force. Instead, self-discipline, doing the right thing by G0d, everyone, and everything, and doing actions of lovingkindness is the driving force.

A human being who is smart and might be involved in any type of professional career can be living primarily as either the G0dly or animal Soul. True wisdom, though, will only be experienced and reside in those who live as their Divine Soul. We all have the choice of which Soul to follow. If the higher existence is desired, the journey there can only be accomplished through the hard work and discipline required to refine oneself. Following the animal Soul takes no work or discipline.

Choosing to live the easy path of the animal Soul and chasing your physical desires without temperance exposes you to potential addiction of all sorts as well as mental and physical health problems. Now that you know the source of your drives and what your choices are, the wise choice is to decide to live the identity of your Divine Soul. How do you go about accomplishing that? You have to have a path for actualizing, knowing, strengthening, and growing your Divine Soul while at the same time doing something to constain the opposing animal Soul.

You have two options to handle your animal Soul. The first is to attempt to eliminate and negate it by only allowing thought, speech, and action generated by the Divine Soul and ignoring and stopping that of the animal Soul. This process can be a monumental task requiring hard work and strict self-discipline. The other option is to transform the Animal Soul into a helpmate for the Divine Soul. This is done by taking the strong impulsive unrestrained drive for bodily pleasure and transforming this powerful energy through intention, hard work, and discipline, into service of the mission of the Divine Soul.

Ultimately, regardless of the path you choose, success over your animal Soul requires strict "actions of inaction." This translates to "just say no." Your brain is above your heart while standing or sitting and this is an easy reminder that you must use your brain to temper your heart. You must train your brain to rule over your heart. Your Divine Soul must control your brain with wisdom and monitor and overrule any and all potential temptation by your animal Soul and its influence over your heart and emotions.

The heart and emotions are about how you feel about something. These feelings are generally short term responses to potentially complex problems that require long term solutions. Our best choices in life are not made when we live by rushed emotional reactions expressed with our thought, speech, or action. Rather they result from tempering our emotions with well thought out and measured long term intellectual and wise responses.

More:

For some humor about struggling with one's identity and split personalities, the comedian, Jackie Mason, has told a joke about going to the psychiatrist to find out who he is. He starts, "I now know who I am. But there was a time that I didn't know who I was. It's a lucky thing my psychiatrist told me who I am. He told me that I was not my real self. He said, "This is not you." So, I asked, "If it's not me, then who is it? Is it you?" He answered, "No, it's not me either." So, I said, "Then who is it?" The psychiatrist said, "I don't know." So, I responded, "Then what do I need you for?" The psychiatrist said, "I'm here to help you look for the real you and find out who you are. Together we're going to look for the real you." I responded, "If I don't know who I am, how do I know who to look for? And even if I find me, how do I know that it's the real me? If I want to look for me, why do I need you? I can look for me by myself. Or I can take my friends. We know where I was. We'll know where to look. Besides, what if I find the real me and he's even worse than me? Why do I need him? I don't make enough money for myself. Do I need a partner? Ten years ago, I would have been glad to look for anybody. Now that I'm doing good, why should I look for him? If he needs help, let him look for me."

The psychiatrist said, "Your appointment is over. The search for the real you will have to continue at your next appointment, and that will be $200 please." He then thought to himself, "If this is not the real me, why should I give him the $200? I'll look for the real me and let him give the psychiatrist the $200. What if I find the real me and he doesn't think it's worth $200? Then I'm stuck giving my money for the real me for nothing. For all I know, the real me is going to a different psychiatrist altogether. He might even be a psychiatrist himself." I said to the psychiatrist, "Wouldn't it be funny if you're the real me and you owe me $200? Tell you what, I'll charge you $100 and we'll call it even."

9

Now Be Ready to Eat a Wholesome Soulful

We have discussed what we need to do to conquer our animal Soul. A large part of this venture requires strong identification as the Divine Soul. The path to identifying as the Divine Soul is a challenging one. This is especially so because of the heavily marketed superficial outer appearance orientation based on the belief that "seeing is believing" and the prevalence of mirrors. This focus on appearance rather than content is held by many of our parents and families, our teachers, our healthcare providers, marketers, and society and culture generally. Since the Soul is nonphysical, invisible, and contained within and hidden by the body, it is often given too little attention with resultant lack of awareness and knowledge of its existence, function, relationships, and capabilities.

In the life of a human being the body feeds, grows, gives off waste, and is active. Optimally, you as the Divine Soul also feed, grow, give off waste, and make things happen. The Divine Soul is thought to be an infinitesimally tiny piece of G0d and is described as resulting from the breath of G0d dating back to the creation of Adam, the first man. Our very limited knowledge of the infinitely complex G0d is the reason for use of an anthropomorphic description of the creation of humankind. G0d is described as having inserted His "breath" by "blowing" into the already molded body of Adam which was fashioned from some combination of earth, dirt, and clay.

We can analogize and consider G0d to be not only the Creator and Ultimate Cause for the existence of everything, but also "the Everything." Just as each of us is a Soul in a body, G0d is kind of like the Soul and body of the whole universe. In fact, the word universe etymologically consists of uni- and -verse. Uni- is one and -verse usually refers to a sentence in the bible. The first sentence of the Torah or bible in English is, "In the beginning G0d created the heavens and the earth." The heavens and the earth comprise the entire physical world which might be thought of as the "body of G0d" and is known as the universe. We are like G0d and are said to be created in the "image of G0d."

Each of us is a small piece of G0d, the Soul, housed in a body, just as G0d might be said to be the Soul of the world contained within the body of the world. However, whereas our existence is finite and our comprehension of G0d is minimal, G0d is infinitely infinite in every way. Everything that exists is sustained and created anew by G0d in every new moment. We are totally dependent on G0d for our lives, sustenance, healing, and the world we live in.

Sustenance of the Divine Soul is provided by Soul nutrition or Soul Food. Soul Food is any thought, speech, or action that connects the Divine Soul with G0d. Love and fear of G0d and faith in God are important components of Soul Food. An analogy to help understand our need to connect with G0d is provided by a raindrop or a piece of sand. A solitary raindrop or grain of sand alone has very little substance or value. But when the raindrop is part of a cloud or the ocean, and the piece of sand is part of the seashore, their real purpose is actualized. Similarly, a solitary Divine Soul on its own, not connected to anything more significant than itself, is isolated and lonely and will have limited ability to fulfill its purpose and mission. It will be hungry for connection. In the absence of connection there is an emptiness and a natural yearning to connect.

The Divine Soul is a separated tiny piece of G0d that yearns to join with G0d and other Divine Souls. But our physical world presents infinitely many choices, diversions, and distractions for us humans to connect with and even worship. Bodily pleasure, skillful marketing, and our own self-delusion can trick us into believing that transient temporal things we connect with are worthwhile and meaningful. We can delude ourselves into thinking G0d is not real, and that G0d has no place in our lives. But G0d was always, is always, and will always be. G0d is our cloud, our ocean, our sandy beach, our Rock.

Without purposeful thought, speech, and action to draw close, connect, and bond with G0d, our Divine Soul will always feel disconnected, unfulfilled, and empty. Lack of G0d in our lives leaves a vacuum that can only be filled with G0d. Substituting anything else for G0d connection is like filling up the gas tank with water or oil instead of gas. You won't be able to get where you need to go. You will continue to exist, but you won't truly be living the life you are meant to live.

The Divine Soul is incomplete by itself. It is at best a half of a whole. This concept is analogous to saying everyone always has a broken heart and one of the ongoing goals of life is for us to work to complete and fill our hearts. The Divine Soul and heart have many options for connection. The primary connection is G0d. Ultimately, we can form many fifty-fifty half-shekel relationships and connections to fulfill our lives. It is most important to choose one's connections and relationships carefully, and it is equally important to prioritize them wisely.

Soul Hunger for G0d and for healthy connections and relationships affects the brain, the heart, and the stomach. If unsatisfied, Soul Hunger causes emptiness, loneliness, and pain. Living only in the physical leaves you no choice but to eat food to satisfy your sense of hunger. But no type or amount of physical food will satisfy Soul Hunger. The result is an endless cycle of unfulfilled eating and weight gain. Therein lies the prime cause of the worldwide obesity epidemics plaguing adults and children. People have left G0d out of their lives thinking this is a rational choice. A human life without connection to G0d is like the raindrop staying as a raindrop, never to join the clouds or oceans, and the grain of sand remaining isolated, never to join the seashore. These are metaphors for a lonely, disconnected, and unfulfilled existence. Soul Hunger is the outcome.

Getting yourself on track to solve this dilemma requires some degree of knowledge of the existence of your Divine Soul and of G0d. You must be willing to check it out. Your Divine Soul must desire Ultimate Truth-the Highest Truth possible. This truth is above all science and all of our learned subjects and all of our physical endeavors and creations. What is science? It is our limited and flawed ability through trial and error to unravel various truths. In many areas, scientists can unravel how things work and reveal truths that we might otherwise not think to explore. However, scientists are generally trained in the science of things and not in G0d or the nonphysical Divine Soul.

The Truth we must seek includes much of science yet towers far above it, such that the science unraveled by the scientists is but the "shadow" cast by G0d on the world. If we might use an iceberg to represent G0d, science is but the tip of the iceberg and addresses only the small bit that the scientists are privileged to see and misses the predominant edifice that is hidden to the eye. Science is always in a state of flux. "Old truths" are frequently relegated to the dustbin of history and are replaced by "new truths."

Soul Food, first and foremost, recognizes that human life is unfulfilled and never complete without a relationship with G0d. This awareness is a matter of faith without which we may experience discontentment, unfulfillment, emptiness, loneliness, and hunger. The Soul Hunger is for understanding that you are the Divine Soul and for G0d. As this new identity, you are a piece of G0d and have the newfound responsibility of respecting yourself, G0d, and all of G0d's creations. Your new mission is to do everything in your power to connect with G0d, and selflessly serve G0d.

The Soul Food that all humans crave is any thought, speech, and action that brings one closer to G0d, thereby fostering greater depth of G0dly understanding, meaning, and purpose. Aligning one's thought, speech, and action with G0d and the service of G0d nourishes and fortifies the Divine Soul. Learning to develop this kind of relationship with G0d can be accomplished in a variety of ways. Reading and learning G0dly wisdom on your own or with a partner, group, or class with help from authentic teachers is an invaluable source of Soul Food. Speaking words of G0dly wisdom and lovingkindness to uplift those around you, performing acts of lovingkindness, and actualizing your existence as Divine Soul and Human Being are more nourishment for the Soul.

"Human Being" is both a noun and a verb. The descriptive verb we are looking for here is Being G0dly by performing and seeking out actions of lovingkindness. Our mission as human beings is really to be acts of lovingkindness. These actions include respecting and honoring parents, caring for the widow, orphan, and those too challenged to be able to care for themselves, and living as a G0dly role model for all to see including children and adults. Displaying lovingkindness also means readily giving of yourself to those less fortunate, whether kind uplifting words, a simple greeting, a mere smile or twinkle in your eye, a monetary gift, food, clothing, housing, transportation, your time, or any other helpful thing. It is vital to remember that in all you do you are serving as a teacher to all who can see or hear you. In that role, you should always attempt to uplift and "light up" those around you with G0dly wisdom, and whatever you do, please try to avoid leading others astray by "placing a stumbling block before the blind."

In our modern world, professionals are trained to be "sharks" in medicine, law, business, and many other careers. Profit motive is generally the shark food rather than being kind and doing the right thing. It can be easier and often second nature to follow the shark dictates of the profession and occupation rather than exhibiting real concern for the patient or client. Blindly applying the tunnel vision principles of the trade for profit motive to people who are innocently ignorant regarding their health, law, or business, etc. can be detrimental to them.

Instead of using your career for profit motive alone and "placing a stumbling block before the blind," consider the plight of the human being seeking your help, and work with them to determine the best personalized solution for their problem. The Soul is nourished by seeking out the deliberate G0dly way rather than the shark's way. Perhaps we would be better served by replacing the selfish "shark mentality" with a kind altruistic "tuna mentality." Soul Food as thought, speech, and action can be found and enjoyed as part of your regular daily existence. You do not have to disappear to a monastery. Be patient with yourself and allow for a gradual process of growth and transformation.

More:

Sometimes in life we look to others for help in our daily lives. We typically respect professionals and their knowledge of their chosen disciplines of law, medicine, business, etc. Yet, in our search for answers and truth, it is sometimes difficult to know who is truly helping us and guiding us on the right path and who might be taking advantage of us. The following story is about fashioning our actions and services to truly fit the needs of others and thereby demonstrate lovingkindness, rather than putting patients, clients, and fellow humans "in a box" to have them serve whatever selfish needs the professionals may have.

There was a poor young man with limited resources who was engaged to be married to the love of his life. He went to a local tailor to have a suit made for his wedding. The tailor assured him that he would work around his limited means and everything would be fine. He had the groom come in to measure first for his shirt. When it was finished, and he came in to try it on, the neck was too tight, one sleeve was too long, and the other was too short. He complained to the tailor. The tailor told him to stiffen his neck, pull one arm in and stretch the other one out. He told him everything would be fine. The young man had trouble comprehending this, but he innocently trusted the tailor. Why shouldn't he? He was, of course, the tailor, and he certainly must have known what he was doing.

Then he was measured for his pants, and when he came back to try them on, he ran into the same dilemma. The waist was too tight, one pant leg was too long and one too short. Again, he complained to the tailor, and yet the tailor told him all was okay. He was told to hold in his stomach, stretch out one leg and pull in the other leg by tilting his pelvis and low back. He did what the tailor said, and although this whole process seemed very strange to him, he trusted the tailor and his expertise.

Next, the groom came to be measured for the jacket, and when he came back to try it on, one arm was too long, and one was too short. The tailor again reassured him. He then tried on the shirt, pants, and jacket. The tailor helped him to contort his body to make the suit look good. The groom was puzzled, but at last he had his wedding suit. He trusted the tailor, and anyway, he didn't have the time or money to do anything different.

When the day of the wedding came, all the guests were assembled in the wedding hall. Everyone was anticipating a lovely wedding with a beautiful bride and groom. When the groom entered the hall in his new suit holding his body in a contorted position to make the suit look good, everyone reacted the same way. They were shocked. They didn't understand why he looked so deformed. They concluded that since he was so deformed, he must have had a brilliant tailor to have somehow made such a well-fitting suit.

Recognizing lovingkindness can be a simple and moving experience, especially when the act of kindness is genuine. There are other times when profit motive biases built into our systems allow professionals to seem to be the best and seem to be serving others' needs, but like "the emperor has no clothes" and "the wizard of oz," the truth is not always what it seems. It is truly shameful when trained, educated professionals who are supposed to be in the business of helping the public instead "place stumbling blocks before the blind." These culprit professionals are so skilled at what they do that they often go undetected.

10

A Spiritual Life

S oul Food nourishes the Divine Soul. Physical food nourishes the body.
Providing nourishment for only the Soul or only the body misses the
mark and can have untoward consequences including illness and even
untimely death. A delicate balance of nourishing both Soul and body is
required to accomplish our purpose and mission.

The word in everyday use today to express the nonphysical Soul aspect
of one's life is "spiritual." People commonly state that they don't believe
in G0d and are not religious, but that they are very spiritual. When they
talk about their spiritual endeavors, they describe meditation, yoga, going
to the beach or mountains, or just breathing, etc.

"Spiritual" is a fascinating word. It has etymological components of
"spir-" and "-ritual." "Spir" refers to breathing like in respire, perspire,
expire, aspire, and conspire. "Ritual" connotes something that is repeated
over and over habitually from day to day. Spiritual used to have the common meaning of being connected to G0d through one's daily ritual practices. "Breathing" applied to a ritual means to make that ritual part of
ourselves in the deepest way possible. Spiritual rituals are all meant to be

connections to G0d. Their purpose is to make us better and stronger in our service of G0d and in our lives generally.

Just as we create and practice habitual rituals for feeding our body such as what, where, how, when, and with whom we eat, feeding our Soul is best accomplished by practicing rituals. Feeding your Soul and satisfying Soul hunger is best accomplished with thought, speech, and action that is repeated regularly. Depending on the particular thought, speech, or action, this can mean constant repetition through the day, or at a specific time every day, or at a given time or day in the week, month, or year.

Spiritual Soul Food is best when it is accompanied by purposeful intention to serve G0d. The intention itself serves as Soul Food. Aligning oneself with G0d to be connected just like the raindrop in the ocean is Soul Food. Ultimately, everything we think, say, and do, can be devoted to the service of and connection with G0d. It is all about having the intention to do so. Waking up, showering, brushing teeth, exercising, eating, working, having friends and meeting people, sleeping, etc. can all be accomplished purely for the body to feel good without any notion of G0d. Alternatively, all of these activities and more can be intentionally done for and in the service of G0d.

Living a genuinely spiritual life does not limit our physical capabilities. Rather it enriches a life of bodily physical existence to a life of true living with G0dly connection and service. This spiritual life is Soul Food and provides for a satisfying and happy life without the need to find a false replacement for Soul Food. The Soul Hunger, which otherwise goes un-abated and is never satisfied by endless eating, is very adequately managed by the truly spiritual life.

As we nourish our Divine Soul, it grows and becomes brighter, stronger, and more powerful. This process is facilitated in two ways. Thought, speech, and action that connects with G0d is the nourishing Soul Food we need, and the more we consume, the better. The Divine Soul is similarly fed by eliminating any thought, speech, and action that does not connect with G0d or that distracts or diverts one's attention from G0d. Practically speak-ing, then, the whole of human life boils down to recognizing our Divine

Soul, feeding it, growing It, and removing the unG0dly from it. That's it. One might ask whether this is not a selfish way to approach the world. As we have discussed, intrinsic to the process of progressively developing one's Divine Soul is performing acts of lovingkindness in all our relationships including with other people, G0d, oneself, and animals, plants, and the entire physical world. This process is meant to be anything but selfish.

More:

Different people have developed different interpretations of the words spirit and spiritual. Some have removed any notion of G0d or Soul when using these words. But there is a company that has gone to extreme lengths to put the non-physical concepts of G0d and Soul directly at the heart of their corporate identity and customer service. Spirit Airlines is all about the non-physical. Their flights and airplanes optimize room for G0d and Soul or spirit.

Recognizing the huge importance and significance of G0d and Soul, they leave little room for the physical aspects of our lives like our physical bodies and our stuff. Lack of adequate room for your physical body and possessions may seem uncomfortable at first. However, Spirit is challenging us to experience what it means to abandon our physical connections and instead navigate the nonphysical world and identify as a nonphysical Divine Soul first and foremost. Limiting our bodily and physical entanglements in this way, one can appreciate flying Spirit Airlines. Why else would they call themselves Spirit?

Hopefully you recognize this piece as humorous and sarcastic. If you have flown with Spirit Airlines, you probably realize that they provide some of the most economical flights by limiting space for seating and baggage. Although I doubt that flying with Spirit Airlines is meant to convey any spiritual meaning (then why do they call themselves Spirit?), there is profound relevance to the notion of finding spiritual meaning through challenging experiences.

11

You Are Not What You Eat

It is common knowledge that "you are what you eat." This phrase means that via the process of digestion, selective molecules of food that you eat become incorporated into molecules and cells of your physical body. Of course, the quantity and quality of the food you eat can impact your physical health and well-being. But is this the highest order of understanding of what eating is about? We have discussed how it is possible to live a purely physical life governed by the motto "what you see is what you get." We have also discussed the possibility of living your identity as a Divine Soul, a nonphysical G0dly entity.

We human beings are not the only creations with a Soul. Just as we have a Divine Soul, every creation of G0d has a Soul nature. Minerals have the purest Soul nature, then come herbs, vegetables, and fruits, and last are animals of all types. Minerals, herbs, vegetables, and fruits all have a peaceful Soul nature. Animals are of diverse types with many different kinds of Soul natures. Some are peaceful herbivores, some are carnivores and kill, some attack, some threaten in various ways, some scavenge, some poison, etc. When we eat an animal, we generally are taught to enjoy an excellent pleasurable taste, and some of us are about seeking healthier animal food products. But when did you last hear anyone speak of the Soul nature of the animal you intend to eat?

You, your Divine Soul, are not what you eat. Instead, your Divine Soul becomes, in part, what you don't eat. Since the real you is your nonphysical Divine Soul and not your physical body, the real you, your Divine Soul, cannot be what you physically eat. The Soul nature of the food you eat is nonphysical and is absorbed by your Soul. Ultimately you, the nonphysical Divine Soul, is not what you eat, your physical food, but instead is impacted in part by the Soul nature of your food, what you don't eat.

Those physical foods that have the most elevated Soul natures are the healthiest for the Soul. These are healthy minerals, herbs, fruits, and vegetables, with avoidance of food made from animals of all kinds. If animal food is desired, consider the Soul nature of the animal and whether it is a nature you desire for your Soul. Intention during food shopping and food preparation and eating, eating to maintain a healthy body to better use it in the service of G0d rather than merely eating for bodily pleasure, thanking G0d for a healthy body and for nutritious food before and after eating are all important determinants of who you are as a Divine Soul. You as a Divine Soul are not what you eat. You are what you don't eat. You are your thoughts, speech, and action in the service of G0d.

More:

Once in a far-off land there was a king who was desperately seeking a suitor for his daughter, the princess. Many came from near and far to seek her hand in marriage, but none were suitably qualified by both the king's and the princess's standards. The king decided to force the issue to appeal to his kingdom who were all looking forward one day to the princess's marriage. He declared to all that the next person to enter the palace would automatically become the husband of the princess. Then in walked the gardener of the king's estates.

The gardener was overwhelmed with excitement and joy. He decided he would be the best husband to the princess. He grew all the finest fruits and vegetables and made sure every day to find the very best of everything to bring to his bride. He brought her the very best and tastiest potatoes, tomatoes, and apples. He was pleased with his ability to give her the best. But the finest and best that the farmer had to offer his princess bride were not anywhere near what she was used to and what she expected in marriage.

The princess in this story represents the nonphysical Divine Soul that requires and is accustomed to nourishment from Soul Food of the highest order. Her new husband, the gardener, represents the physical body. He is not functioning on the level of Soul and instead knows how to prepare the best and healthiest physical food. This relationship does not work because they are totally mismatched. Feeding even the best and tastiest of physical food to the Soul does not satisfy the Soul nor Soul Hunger.

Most people the world over think like the gardener. They know how to feed the body with every possible delectable, but they don't know that the princess is from the palace. She is different and only a refined G0dly food will satisfy her. Just as the gardener does not recognize the princess's reality and needs, many people see and think of themselves as a body only and have no conception of Soul. The Soul is from and of G0d and requires special Soul Food.

Soul Food is anything that nourishes and grows the Divine Soul and helps free it from the desires of the animal Soul. Participating in community prayer service can serve as Soul food. But places of worship can be smart and recognize that serving physical food can be a useful method for attracting congregants. Some worshippers show up more for bodily food than for prayerful Soul Food. One morning after prayer worship and fellowship two older congregants were talking together, and one asked the other what he thought of the prayer service that morning. He replied that the food was excellent, but the service was awful.

The humor in this joke involves the distinctions between the nonphysical world of the Soul and the physical world of the body. The food discussed in the joke is a double entendre and can refer to both Soul Food related to the prayer service as well as the physical food that was served.

The use of the word "service" represents a second double entendre and adds to the humor because it can refer to both the prayer service and the food service. We always are granted the opportunity to be positive and uplifting and make the best of every situation. When it comes to the food, whether Soul Food or physical food, and to the service of prayer or to food service, pleasing everyone is an extremely difficult task requiring great skill.

12

What Role Does
Exercise Play?

Any discussion of obesity with the hope of solving this worldwide
epidemic problem cannot limit itself to food alone. Another critical
consideration is the activity and level of energy expenditure so that
the calories consumed from food are burned off. Exercise or fitness are
the general terms used to refer to this activity. If we consider the components of our Soul and body, and we are looking to maintain or achieve
optimal good health for each component, a better understanding of what
we should do becomes clear. We have defined the human being as a nonphysical Divine Soul housed in a physical body which has an intrinsic
Animal Soul.

The key functional parts of the body are the brain, the heart, and other
organ systems including nervous, cardiovascular, pulmonary, musculoskeletal, sensory, digestive, genitourinary, reproductive, and skin. When discussing obesity and weight loss, exercise and fitness are generally meant to
refer to bodily activity involving the heart and the muscles and joints. But

the specific need that we all have for ourselves as a whole organism, for Soul and body, as well as for all our component parts is Motion or Movement.

Obesity and weight gain are obviously associated with a lack of self-control and discipline with one's mouth. Additionally, there is a huge association of obesity with the ubiquitous human Sedentary Lifestyle. Every human being, regardless of their level of activity or how much exercise they do, lives a Sedentary Lifestyle. Evaluation of everyone's twenty-four-hour day would reveal that the large majority of time is spent sitting in a variety of different types of chairs, another large amount of time is spent lying down, and an additional period is spent standing. What is common to sitting, lying down, and standing is a total lack of physical motion. This lack of motion is considered by some to be a cause of obesity as well as a result of obesity. And obesity is but one health epidemic comprising what is known as Sedentary Disease.

The number one killer, cause of pain and suffering, and healthcare cost is Sedentary Disease. Sedentary Disease is caused by our Sedentary Lifestyle and includes a collection of epidemic diseases. These are obesity, low back pain, heart disease, atherosclerosis, hypertension, diabetes, depression, cancer, and muscle, tendon, bone, and joint ailments that occur with aging. Senile Dementia and Alzheimer's Disease have also been included as Sedentary Disease and attributed to our Sedentary Lifestyle.

An essential tool to help prevent weight gain and obesity and all the epidemic diseases of Sedentary Disease is Motion. Life is motion. Lack of movement or stasis leads to sclerosis and death. All of our human parts require motion for a healthy life. The Divine Soul, the Animal Soul, the brain, heart, lungs, blood vessels, muscles and joints, as well as all of our organ systems each require their own vitalizing motion for healthy sustenance. This motion needs to be part of the regular diet for Soul and body.

Motion for the Divine Soul means a constant feeding of the Soul and growth of the Soul with concomitant jettisoning of any unG0dly thought, speech, and action. Motion for the Animal Soul means an ongoing process of controlling, limiting, and harnessing its drive, or transforming its drive and energy into service of the Divine Soul. Motion for the brain and intellect means frequent use of the brain by the Divine Soul to control, develop, and create G0dly thought, speech, and action. Conceptually this motion of the brain would be preventive of stasis and sclerosis of the brain and concomitant senile dementia and Alzheimer's Disease.

Motion for the heart is twofold involving both emotions and serving as the physical engine of the body. The word emotion interestingly contains the word motion. As human beings we experience many emotions. These emotions are generally short-term reactions to life experiences, and they require temperance by the Divine Soul and brain. Our primary emotion and driving force should be love for G0d and the desire to connect with G0d. When other emotions occur which often can be troubling and painful and get in the way, it is important for our Soul and brain to focus on our Soul Diet of G0dly thought, speech, and action. Swift movement of toxic emotions out of the heart is thereby facilitated and it can once again be filled with love.

Motion for the heart doesn't just refer to the emotions. The heart is also the key physical component or engine of the cardiopulmonary vascular system, which consists of the heart, lungs, and blood vessels. It is a scientific wonder in that it is an alive perpetual machine that pumps nonstop each moment of every human being's life. The heart pumps our life's oxygen-carrying blood through our entire body to every cell via the vascular tree of blood vessels including the arteries and veins. Oxygen is the primary nutrient that we thrive on and that every cell needs to survive. Our lungs are responsible for the delivery of oxygen to our bloodstream. Heart disease including myocardial infarction, congestive heart failure, and coronary artery disease, atherosclerosis, and hypertension are well known common afflictions involving the heart and blood vessels. Good physical health mandates good health of our heart, lungs, and blood vessels.

Aerobic or cardiopulmonary vascular exercise is life-preserving and is our most important physical exercise and should be done on a frequent regular basis. Walking, jogging, bicycling, swimming, rollerblading, basketball, and tennis are examples of healthy aerobic exercise that will challenge the heart, lungs, and blood vessels and increase heart strength.

The second most important type of exercise for good physical health is muscle and joint stretching. During our lifetime, five significant bodily changes occur that tend to result in shortening, stiffening, and tightening of our muscles and joints resulting in pain and stiffness. First, when we are young, we are mostly water content on a cellular level, and as we age, this water content decreases. Second, when we are young the tissues are supple and fluid, and as we age, they become stiff and immobile, similar to the comparison of the flexibility of the branch of a sapling to the branch of an old grown tree.

Third, we are bombarded nearly constantly with stress energies from our interpersonal relationships, finances, almost nonstop interaction with the multiple functions of our ever-present cell phones, job duties, car driving, and living. Just as a rubber-band absorbs energy when stretched and that energy is realized when the rubber-band is let go and it flies through the air, our muscles and ligaments readily absorb stress energies. When the muscles and ligaments absorb energy they contract, thereby shortening, stiffening, and tightening. The heart and stomach are both large muscles, and along with the muscles and ligaments of the joints, are the constant target of ever-present stress energies. Regular optimal muscle and joint movement can release this energy, promote health, and prevent pain and stiffness. Fourth, muscle and ligament injuries incurred along life's journey generally involve stretching, tearing, and bleeding of the tissue. The mechanism of healing that we are endowed with results in the formation of fibrous scar tissue rather than new muscle tissue. This scar tissue is stiff, tight, and shortened, and the way to promote its optimal function is to stretch it regularly and maximally.

Fifth, when we are young, we tend to be more physically active, and when we age, we become sedentary. Living a sedentary life, we tend to assume certain bodily positions for prolonged periods. Over many years, our muscles and ligaments will tend to shorten, stiffen, tighten, and they can even calcify in the position of maximum motion or the position they are habitually kept in.

People participate in all kinds of fitness programs for exercise, including yoga, Pilates, tai chi, aerobics, Zumba, and spinning. However, none of these activities offers a clear, focused, simple to perform, wisdom-based, head to toe muscle and joint, full range of motion program. After aerobic cardiac exercise, a total body full range of motion program is the next most essential healthy physical exercise we need. Regular full range of motion is important for healthy balance and fall prevention. This exercise is extremely important to stem the tide of falls in the elderly, which is associated with a very high rate of morbidity and mortality.

The third type of exercise we can pursue is not nearly as important as the first two, yet it is often the first category of exercise, and sometimes the only exercise many people pursue. As we have discussed, many people are focused on what they see of themselves in the mirror, and to lose weight and tone muscles, they pursue a strengthening program using free weights or exercise machines in a gym. The prevalence of gyms with free weights and circuits of strengthening machines throughout the United States is wonderful and has helped fuel the desire to strengthen muscles. But for overall physical health, this is not option one or two and comes in at a distant third.

Exercise in any gym or with any trainer should be undertaken with care to improve one's overall health, wellness, and fitness, and not incur injury or harm. Each individual has their own specific makeup, capability, and history, and therefore, exercise programs need to be personalized to be safe. Many personal trainers in gyms and elsewhere are young and are trained to deal with healthy young clients. However, many people who are aging and have a history of injury, accident, surgery, and other problems also participate in gyms and fitness programs. Often the trainers and gyms do not have the training or experience to address these problems. By simply doing what everyone else in the gym is doing with the various machines and exercises, certain people will be causing themselves harm and injury. Care must be taken to understand one's limitations before undertaking an exercise program and to make sure the program is personalized to oneself.

A healthy exercise program can go a long way towards reducing Soul Hunger and improving physical health and fitness. Most important is a program of regular aerobic exercise to strengthen heart, lungs, blood vessels, and the rest of the body as a life-saving measure. The next most vital component is a regular total body muscle and joint full range of motion program to enable muscle and joint health, overall body function, and sturdy and stable balance. The last component to include in one's exercise program is a strengthening program to help maintain and improve bodily strength and function. Ideally your exercise program should be personalized to your specific station in life, your overall health, your history of medical conditions, injuries, and surgeries, your heart, lung, and vascular status, your neurological and muscular status, your posture and balance, and your limb and joint status.

Patients with muscle and joint pain tend to be frequent flyers and bottleneck emergency rooms. Emergency room providers would like to devote their time to true emergencies rather than the common low back, neck, knee, shoulder, and other pain patients. A solution to this healthcare problem might be to educate an advanced group of trainers in the ramifications of pain, injury, and surgery so they would know how to manage these types of clients. Then, many people presenting with pain to hospitals and doctors could instead go to gyms and trainers. With proper training and education, the gyms and trainers could be optimized as the best resource for all of these people, provide better care and recovery for those in pain and with injuries, and free up hospital emergency rooms.

More:

There once was a rabbi who would spend hours visiting individually with hundreds to thousands of his followers in his study. People would come from near and far to share their hopes, dreams, and problems with the rabbi and ask him for a personal blessing for themselves and their loved ones. Generally, the only exercise the rabbi would get was on walks to visit members of the community, attend meetings, and visit orphans, widows, the needy, and the sick. But after a long night of one on one sessions with so many of his followers, there would always be a pile of soaking wet clothes on the floor.

Everyone knew this story about the rabbi, but the question everyone had was, "What was the meaning of the pile of soaking wet clothes?" There is a heartwarming and straightforward explanation. When a visitor initially presented to the rabbi and shared their story, the rabbi was listening in his clothes. He had to interpret and understand the profound meaning on the level of the Soul, intellect, and emotions of the visitor including any pain they might be experiencing. To truly know him, the rabbi would symbolically remove his own wet clothes and put on those of the visitor. Once he knew him, he would take off the wet visitor's garments and put back a set of his own dry clothes to be able to advise and bless the visitor successfully and adequately.

This process of two changes of clothes or garments whereby the rabbi would go through three sets of garments for each visitor, each time working up a sweat in dealing with the personal issues at hand as well as the exercise associated with the repetitive "physical change of clothes" was part of the rabbi's self-assigned job. It was about doing his best in the service of G0d, his community, and every visitor. The rabbi didn't want to leave any stone unturned and did not want to "place a stumbling block before the blind." To genuinely help another, it is very important to first understand their problem from their perspective and remove one's personal biases. "Don't judge a man until you've walked in his shoes."

The rabbi in this story apparently got a good physical workout, and even drenched his clothes, from hours spent switching roles from his own to that of his visitors. He did many symbolic garment changes that represented his sincere effort to understand the visitor completely and then to give the best advice. Although this exercise is not typical of gym fitness, this is an exercise activity worthy of any public servant, especially professionals working in the public trust, including doctors, lawyers, and businessmen. Perhaps if sincere and greater effort and time were made to get to know and help others, we would experience less stress and pain, less exercise would be needed, and we would generally be healthier with less disease.

13

The Pearl and the Oyster

Conquering pain necessitates a "box of tools" or a "Pain Toolbox" to use against pain. Our Pain Toolbox includes our diet paradigm, including living one's identity as a Divine Soul, connecting with G0d, and selflessly serving G0d with G0dly, health-promoting, and wholesome thought, speech, and action. All of the various products and services offered by MISSING LINKS HEALTH, INC. are especially created by me to be part of your Pain Toolbox. These include this book, SITFIT CHAIR-a total body gym in a portable multi-positional and multi-functional chair, 1 MINUTE STRETCH-a course teaching a medically essential head to toe muscle and joint full range of motion stretching routine, STRETCHING FOR PAIN RELIEF-a forty video course teaching how to optimize muscle and joint health and fitness, and MRI-MED-SURG DISRUPT-A consulting platform focusing on the flaws and fixes in the development and utilization of MRI to determine surgical planning.

At the heart of the Toolbox is the understanding of how a pearl is formed because this process has much to teach us humans about how we handle our pain. A pearl is created by an oyster in response to pain. When a painful irritant enters the oyster, the oyster doesn't change. Human beings, on the other hand, typically react to pain with a behavioral change that is generally a change for the worse. We become silent, reticent, sad, depressed, upset, suicidal, abusive of and addicted to various substances, angry, argumentative, combative, and sometimes go on a rampage murdering at work or school. In contradistinction, the oyster does not change but instead secretes a substance that surrounds and walls off the painful irritant and then repeats this process over and over, creating concentric layers until a beautiful pearl is formed.

Applying all the tools from our Pain Toolbox and diet paradigm will entrust the person confronted with pain with the ability to turn that pain into beautiful pearls. No longer do we have to experience uncontrolled toxic emotional reactions to our pain. No longer do we have to suffer unnecessarily. Some people carry pain around with them as a comfort or as a familiar "buddy." They have become so accustomed to it that they can't imagine what their life would be like or what they would do without it. Our toolbox empowers us to better understand and manipulate pain rather than having to surrender to it.

The spherical concentrically layered anatomy of the pearl is analogous to the process of concentric layering and development of our own human lives. Each concentric ring can represent habitual thought processes, speech, and action that we make part of ourselves. In our lives, the more we repeat a thought, speech, or action, the thicker the layer. We can add layers, grow layers, and remove layers. This concentric ring model is analogous in many ways to the cross-sectional rings of the tree.

In dealing with pain, the longer it's cause persists, the more troubled the afflicted person may become, and the more difficult and more time it will take to resolve the pain. The formation of a pearl demonstrates a model for an alternative process. As the oyster confronts the painful irritant, over time the pearl grows layer by layer, gradually bigger and bigger, becoming more and more beautiful and precious. With the right tools, the struggle of dealing with pain can lead to a stronger Divine Soul identity, greater connection with G0d, and the ability to find increased meaning and purpose in life like never before. In this way we too, like the oyster, can transform pain into pearls.

How I came to understand the lessons of the pearl is a personal story. First, my last name is Pearlstein. When I accepted my life's mission to solve my mother's pain, and pain generally, I simultaneously sought out the meaning of my last name. Pearlstein means "stone of pearl" which might connote a very strong, solid, or distinctive pearl. From there I sought to understand how a pearl is formed and learned the relationship of the pearl to pain. Once I learned this lesson of the pearl, I combined my last name, Pearlstein, with my mother's maiden name which is Yagid in Hebrew or Jaget in English. Yagid means "to speak." The combined meaning of these two names, Pearlstein and Yagid, is to speak about the deep mystical lesson of the pearl, and this has become my life's mission along with the creation of the tools of our Pain Toolbox to help transform pain to pearls of wisdom and joy.

Another persistent message for me regarding pearls was that my sweet, sensitive mother enjoyed wearing a string of white pearls around her neck more than any other jewelry. There was something about pearls that gave my mother a simple, pure, joyful pleasure and I remember her wearing them modestly, yet elegantly, and she looked so beautiful. I needed to find a deeper meaning for this joy to close the circle of my understanding of how to turn our pain into pearls. Worn around my mother's neck in the form of a pearl necklace was the symbolic answer to so much pain.

More:

I have a good friend who is a business consultant. Many years ago, he invited me to his office, and he shared one of his business concepts with me. He explained that the rings of the cross-section of a tree are a good organizational model for structuring a business and how it allows for a simple process of putting layers on for growth or removing layers for downsizing. I was already familiar with the tree as a model for humankind.

A tiny seed can grow into a large blooming tree that keeps on growing and some are fruit-bearing. We humans also start conception as a small seed and whereas our bodies can grow to a limited size and height, the Soul is capable of growing, flourishing, and bearing fruit indefinitely, just like the tree. For the seed to successfully become a tree it must be planted in the ground, it disintegrates before it stimulates the soil to allow growth, it needs adequate clean water, exposure to sunlight is crucial, and G0d's blessings will help provide added essential nourishment for growth and life. The process of human growth and development has similar requirements.

Tempering of ambition to grow and succeed with humility is like planting in grounded-being grounded. Decomposition of the seed is our ability to transform old embedded ways, habits, and preconceived notions to a new fresh outlook with accompanying behavioral change. Sunlight for us is G0d's light-the path and direction of truth and goodness. G0d's blessings are achieved be our seeking out G0d, connecting with G0d, and having and building our faith. The ability of a tiny seed to become a fruit-bearing tree capable of producing a great abundance of fruit in its lifetime is analogous to our ability to become a producer of an abundance of acts of lovingkindness in our lifetime, each with its own potential explosive effect in magnifying and spreading lovingkindness and goodness around the world.

We must stay connected to the roots for proper nourishment and life. Stability of the tree in difficult times is more related to the reach and depth of the roots rather than the appearance of the tree above ground. A tree can make beautiful fruit but once the fruit is disconnected from the tree and roots it will die. The lesson for man is to be grounded in truth, balance, and wholeness throughout one's life.

The concept of the rings of the tree added another level of understanding in that each ring represents the type of annual growth the tree experienced. A good year with adequate sunlight, water, and fertilizer would produce a healthy broad ring. A bad year with poor availability of sunlight, water, and fertilizer and maybe with insect infestation would produce a narrow, mottled, and unhealthy ring. This ring model also works for personal transformation in our own lives and the lesson is to avoid bad influences and habits and seek beneficial ones.

Subsequently I found that the onion and onion-skinning offer a similar model of concentric rings which instead of only being a two-dimensional planar cross-section is a three-dimensional spherical model. The message is the same but with an emotional touch. The scent of the onion causes tearing. Tears generally represent pain or joy. The onion connects us to these emotions and sensitivities by making us cry.

The tree and the onion are both good symbols for personal transformation, but neither is as impactful as another naturally occurring ring model which unbeknownst to me was right "under my nose." At a certain time in my life when I sought to understand the derivation and meaning of my last name, Pearlstein, I simultaneously bumped into the deep meaning of the pearl. The pearl is formed as a response to pain. The concentric rings of the tree, onion, and pearl each mark a chronological process of change. Human beings all grow and change.

The pearl ultimately became my choice to convey the concept of personal transformation and how this process occurs on the level of the Soul and is generally triggered by pain. The oyster's ability to transform pain into a beautiful pristine pearl without bringing harm or self-sacrifice to itself is the key to unlock our own healthy process of personal transformation to conquer physical, emotional, and spiritual pain.

14

Justice, Righteousness, Lovingkindness, Holiness

As human beings we can choose how we live our lives. The simplest, natural way to live, requiring little effort, is to continue life after infancy as no more than a big infant living as the Animal Soul, selfishly pursuing pleasureful bodily desires. The higher order of living is to actualize one's identity as the Divine Soul and selflessly devote one's life to the service of G0d. This mission is accomplished through purposeful thought, speech, and action governed by intention, hard work, and self-discipline. The building blocks to create a meaningful life with meaningful fulfilling relationships are justice, righteousness, lovingkindness, and holiness.

Justice is the foundational building block necessary for all of our relationships. The potential relationships and connections in your life include your Soul and body relationship, your relationships with all people, your relationship with G0d, and your relationship with animals, plants, and all other material things. Justice is often thought to be punishment for breaking the law. But justice is the responsibility to "do no harm." Justice means having self-discipline and closing our brains, mouths, and bodies off to thoughts, speech, and actions which might be harmful to any of our relationships. Justice is mostly about avoiding actions which will cause problems and choosing more preferable actions instead. These are actions of inaction, and are enabled by the admirable and honorable strength, courage, and ability in many cases and situations to "just say no." Don't think it, don't speak it, and don't do it. This process allows us to nurture all of our healthy relationships.

Righteousness is the second essential building block that all of our relationships depend on for healthy growth. Righteousness is about fulfilling obligations mandated by our various associations. We should strive to speak appropriately, modestly, and respectfully and do what has to be done in our various relationships. We have obligations to G0d, ourselves, our spouse, our parents, our children, widows, orphans, the needy, the community, strangers, everyone, and everything including animals, plants, and the rest of the material world and the environment.

Lovingkindness is the next building block. One cannot be a loving person without first being just and righteous. If one is not just or righteous, then they are not exemplifying lovingkindness. If one is just and righteous and selflessly gives more in their relationships than is required, with care not to weaken or harm another or their relationship, they are exemplifying lovingkindness.

Holiness is the last building block and requires the incorporation of the first three building blocks of justice, righteousness, and lovingkindness. Holiness goes a step further and is about connecting all one's thoughts, speech, and action to G0d. Holiness mandates knowing that you are the Divine Soul, and your life's mission and purpose is to selflessly serve G0d. It is about separating from and negating any desire to selfishly serve the pleasure of the body and placing one's total faith and life in G0d's hands.

Tackling and accomplishing each of these building blocks takes tough focus and work. It is all about gaining understanding and then applying self-discipline. These building blocks are accessible to everyone and no matter one's place in life, no one is ever too far gone or too late to start building their home, the edifice of their life, with the justice, righteousness, lovingkindness, and holiness building blocks.

More:

There is an old joke that simply says, "In the beginning, G0d created human beings in His own image, and ever since then we have returned the favor." We humans and the religions we develop produce beliefs in which G0d turns out to be very much like us and has the same opinions we have. The journey of personal transformation to better oneself and seek a relationship with G0d needs to be about changing oneself to be more G0dly, and not about changing our notion of G0d to be more like us or to serve us.

A young man who hadn't prayed or been religiously involved before decided he wanted to improve himself by seeking out G0d. He presented to the local house of worship hoping to pray and learn. They told him he wasn't a paying member and, until he was, he couldn't participate. He pleaded with them but ended up home alone, crying his heart out to G0d. Suddenly he heard a voice that said, "My dear son. Please don't feel bad. They don't let me in either." The path toward self-improvement is full of challenges and lessons. Only when you persist in your search for growth will you will find what you seek.

15

Fun, Happiness, and Joy

The driving force in human life is desire. We have seen that desire can be selfless to serve G0d or selfish to serve bodily pleasure. If your goal is to selflessly serve G0d then you must seek out and know what you are needed for. Selfishly serving bodily pleasure is about knowing what your body wants and needs. Knowing and chasing what we are needed for gives us life and health. Selfishly knowing and pursuing what our bodies want and need does not produce life and health. It is said that "I is ill, and we is well" meaning that inward focus on self alone is detrimental, whereas focus on connecting with others and their needs is beneficial. The pleasure that results from our choice of behavior has been described with various words. Fun, happiness, and joy are three of these words.

For some, fun, happiness, or joy are life's goals and the ultimate destination. Fun is one of the most commonly used words in the English language. Everyone wants to know: "Are we having fun?" "Are you going to have fun?" "Is it fun?" "Did you have fun?" The word "fun" is used to mean different things. Sometimes it is used to refer to a family get-together or a meaningful event. I prefer to call these types of events happy or joyous, rather than fun, because "fun" also has a frightening connotation.

When a child rides a rollercoaster, he's having a great time. But when it comes to an end, he often wants to go again, or maybe he cries that he wants to go on a bigger rollercoaster. It's not the rollercoaster that he wants. It's the feeling of the adrenalin that was pumping through his body. He wants more adrenalin and the feeling that comes with it. This aspect of fun is a meaningless transient physical adrenaline kick.

Performers, including comedians, actors, and musicians the likes of John Belushi and Robin Williams, entertain and bring laughter and joy to large audiences. While performing, adrenaline is pumping through their bodies giving them a massive high. This adrenaline high feels better and more exciting than anything else they've ever experienced. But there is a problem in the lives and deaths of John Belushi, Robin Williams, and so many others. The problem is when they go home. At home, there is no audience and no performance. So, there is no adrenaline.

For these performers, the "fun" of adrenaline becomes their substitute for real happiness. At home, without adrenaline, they can feel empty and depressed. Many entertainers have shared their affliction with depression with the public. They don't know what it means to feel happy without adrenaline coursing through their veins, and there was no one to teach them. John Belushi died of a drug overdose, trying to mimic his adrenaline high. Robin Williams committed suicide when he became so afraid that, due to medical issues, he didn't think he could perform well anymore, which was vital to his generation of adrenaline and his adrenaline high.

Without their adrenaline high, many of these performers and many people from all walks of life feel a need to use drugs, many become drug addicts, and many lose or end their lives. They are all seeking fun. Our entire society and culture talk about the experience of fun. But more often than not, the adrenaline high leads to emptiness and depression at home. The desire for fun has helped lead America into a substantial statistical depression. For some time now we have been known as the "Prozac nation."

Happiness is very different from fun and is much less frequently spoken about. Whereas fun is a desire for something that will cause the body to produce adrenaline, happiness has nothing to do with desire. Happiness is about being completely "content with one's lot." That means that absolutely nothing is lacking or needed for happiness. But one's lot is a complicated collection of things consisting of everything going on and every connection in one's life. How can one possibly always be content with so many different things and with many ongoing changes in one's life if this is what would be required to truly achieve happiness?

The trick to true happiness is threefold. The first is to live as the Divine Soul and recognize that everything that exists and that happens is orchestrated by the Creator. Nothing exists or occurs without G0d as the Source. Since everything Created by G0d can only be good and for the good of all, then although things can be a struggle, a challenge, painful, and at times unbearable, they are all for the good. We cannot expect anything to be a certain way just because we are accustomed to it or because it would be good for us. We don't run the world. We are limited in our understanding and cannot fathom G0d's "brain" and why G0d makes or allows things to happen the way they do. The bottom line is that to be happy is to be thankful and feel blessed about everything always.

Second, at any time and at all times in our lives, all we ever have is this present moment. And as soon as we even think of the moment, it is gone. We cannot live in the past, and the future is never guaranteed. At every moment, we must recognize that everything is for the good of all. Our greatest gift after the gift of life is our time. We must realize that every moment is a precious blessing. Once we contemplate how it could have, would have, or should have been, thinking into the past, or how it could, would, or should be, thinking into the future, we are not living in the moment and are sacrificing our ability to be happy. True happiness requires living in the present moment.

The third happiness trick involves an analogy. If you are in a room and it is too hot or too cold you will tweak the thermostat to adjust the temperature. Similarly, we all have a thermostat of mental contentment for anything and everything. Any time a component of your lot changes, whether in your favor or not in your favor, simply adjust your thermostat of mental contentment and say, "I'm okay with that." Of course, you can choose to live with things as they are, or you can pursue any changes you'd like to make. But ultimately happiness requires thanksgiving for and contentment with things as they are at this moment.

To sum up so far, fun is often a transient meaningless physical adrenaline kick. Happiness is first about acknowledging that everything comes from G0d, and therefore everything is for the good of all. Secondly, all we ever have at any time is the present, blessed, precious moment. Thirdly, happiness is a mental thermostat of contentment trick. Fun is physical. Happiness is mental. Whereas this aspect of fun has no redeeming value, happiness is an attribute with great value, worthy of pursuit. Happiness is not an end in itself, but instead is a tremendously useful vehicle to allow us to live meaningful, purposeful lives. When we are happy, we can acknowledge that we are genuinely alive, and a happy life feels better and allows for a more productive life.

Joy is very different from fun and happiness. Joy is the knowledge that you, the Divine Soul, are connected with, and are a part of G0d, at all times. This unbreakable bond should fill you with ultimate glee that you could sing and dance at any moment to acknowledge your strong and meaningful relationship with the Creator. Joy emanates from the Soul, happiness is mental, and fun is physical. Fun is a meaningless transient physical adrenaline kick. Happiness is a mental thermostat of contentment trick. Joy is knowing that you as Divine Soul are intrinsically connected and one with G0d, thereby filling you with the motivation and sense of freedom to sing and dance at any moment.

Our American forefathers were geniuses in their drafting of the Declaration of Independence in which they declared that all human beings are created equal with unalienable rights given to us by our Creator, including preservation of life, liberty, and the pursuit of happiness. They were aware of the need to acknowledge our Creator before even addressing life, liberty, and happiness. They knew we must be thankful to G0d for life. America is blessed to be a democracy in which freedom and liberty are greatly valued. Empowered by G0d and liberty, they recognized the importance of happiness as a powerful vehicle to serve G0d in our earthly purpose and mission. Unlike life and liberty, happiness is not guaranteed. It can be purposely taught and learned, and it can be achieved through life experience and wisdom.

Happiness is not the purpose of life. Instead happiness is the vehicle, tool, or facilitator to allow optimal success in one's endeavors. Happiness is a trained mental attitude that anyone can develop and exhibit at all times. It is a facilitator for peace and balance in one's life. Fun, on the other hand, was not guaranteed or discussed by the forefathers. We would do an excellent service to our forefathers' memory, our country, ourselves, our children, and future generations by being mindful to discontinue and replace the prevalent discussion using the word fun with the words happiness and joy, and by learning to be happy and joyful. Once we possess happiness and joy, a special act of lovingkindness is to share with others.

More:

I always have my different horns in the trunk of my car wherever I go because every time is a good time for music and playing the trumpet. I have a pocket trumpet, regular trumpet, and flugelhorn. Generally, I carry my pocket trumpet in a small black bag over my right shoulder. When I play at a restaurant, bar, or venue of any type, people most commonly see me playing my small pocket trumpet.

Innumerable times people have told me that they have never seen a horn like mine, and they want to know what it is. I've responded by making all kinds of jokes over the years, and lately I answer simply that it's "small." If they prompt me further, I tell them that it's called a pocket trumpet, that the metal tubing is just wound tighter, and that it plays the same as a regular size trumpet. A joke that I often make is that at different times my horn can get bigger. There's always the larger regular trumpet, and larger than that is the flugelhorn. So, I've got interchangeable small, medium, and large horns.

I'm not sure how it happened but explaining my horns and their sizes got me to think about the coffee sizes offered by Starbucks. Everywhere in the world and for all time we have known that there are three basic generic sizes in many things: small, medium, and large. That is until Starbucks had to be different and changed all that.

It has been written that the name Starbucks is derived from the name of Captain Ahab's first mate, Starbuck, in *Moby Dick*. The unique cup size names are said to have evolved from then CEO Howard Schultz's desire to emulate the romance of the Italian coffee bar. Yet, I sense much deeper psychological meaning in the names. I don't think Starbucks is about coffee or donuts or anything that goes in your mouth. It is about making you feel good about yourself and generally happy with yourself. It is playing the role of the master magician by playing a subliminal psychological trick on all who buy Starbucks coffee and products.

Within the corporate name, Starbucks, is everything we are culturally trained to aspire to be and everything we would like to possess. We all would like to be a "star," and we all seek to possess "bucks." The identity and the possession many people dream of are incorporated in the company name and on every store, coffee cup, and other products. They are convincing you that you will have it all at Starbucks and with Starbucks products.

So, what's with the unusual categorization of cup sizes? I think that it is all about you and making you feel good in the material world. It is not about the size of the cup or the amount of coffee. It is about you and your size. We know that there are many short people in the world. Short people generally have lower self-esteem than tall people, and short people do not fare as well in the job and dating markets. So what Starbuck's cup sizes are saying is, "We don't have any small size. At Starbucks, small and short people are not short. Instead, you are magically tall. And now that we have elevated short people to be tall, we can safely and magically make medium and tall people grande. We can do this without embarrassing short people who are now tall. As for extra tall and giant people, that can be embarrassing for everyone else. It is not nice to be immodest and embarrass others, so why not call them by a name that no one recognizes and that really doesn't mean much to most people. We'll call them venti which we've got to go to Latin to understand and find out it means 20, referring to a 20-ounce cup."

This is all marketing. You might feel a sense of more self-esteem and you might feel happy at Starbucks. But be aware that these are feelings about transient materialistic meaningless things. True happiness does not come from outside of you. Being a star, having bucks, wealth, or possessions, or any desirable physical attribute will not guarantee happiness. True happiness is a mental attitude that can only come with experience and wisdom and it only comes from within you. But if you don't mind drinking fifty cents of milk for five dollars, then enjoy Starbucks. Starbucks does generally offer a relaxing environment to do work, and if you are not bothered by the price, you can enjoy their coffee.

The notion that buying Starbucks coffee might bring happiness reminds me of another story. A modern visitor to a laid-back island was relaxing on the beach when he noticed how a fisherman would paddle his boat out to sea each morning to fish for several hours. He would return before noon to sell the fish he caught and then enjoy lunch before taking his daily afternoon nap. The fisherman came back every day with a boatload of fish and was able to sell all of the fish.

The visitor was impressed with the fisherman's success and approached him. He suggested that the fisherman spend the whole day fishing and not just the morning. When the fisherman asked why, the visitor told him he could probably double the money he was making. He told him that he would happily go into partnership with him. They could buy more boats and bigger boats and hire other fisherman. They would be able to catch many boatloads of fish to sell locally and also export.

The fisherman asked what the point of all this extra work was. The visitor told him that he would be able to make so much money that he could eventually just work in the morning, finish by lunch, and nap and relax in the afternoon. The fisherman told him that that's exactly the life he was currently leading, and he was happy with it.

Happiness for the fisherman was about a state of mind and a mental attitude and not about materialistic stuff. The visitor thought he was smarter than the fisherman and tried to teach the fisherman from his perspective. The fisherman was wiser, though, and was at a higher level of thinking. Happiness is about being thankful and content with everything in the current moment. It is not about titles, money, or stuff you may acquire.

16

Life is a Tea Kettle

The tea kettle serves as one model for understanding what human life is about. The components of this model are first, the metal kettle. Second is the fire underneath which we will assume for illustration is a perpetual fire. Third is the water in the kettle which we will assume is in endless supply. Fourth is the resulting steam, and fifth is the kettle spout. The fire represents all of the life changes, challenges, stressors, and sources of energy confronting us at all times day and night 24-7-365, even during sleep. The kettle represents our confining hard physical body along with any physical and nonphysical thought, speech, actions, and things that restrict our ability to "be all we can be." The water in the kettle represents our Divine Soul essence, that nonphysical soft inner G0dly self we all are. The steam represents the transformation of the Soul as it is refined and purified by the ongoing fire.

The spout is open and allows steam to escape freely. If the spout were plugged shut, then the pressure inside the kettle would steadily increase until the weakest link in the metal structure of the kettle would give way and burst. Similarly, in our lives, we can maintain healthy open spouts, which represent our Soul Food and nutrition. These are connecting with

GOd through faith, learning, and prayer, acts of lovingkindness towards other people, GOd, oneself, and animals, plants, and the material world, healthy physical nutrition, healthy exercise, wellness, fitness, and lifestyle, music, living in the present moment, having a positive attitude, and being happy and joyful in all one's relations.

If the fire gets too hot representing our being overwhelmed by stressors, and the techniques for keeping the spout open to release toxic energy are not adequate, then the kettle pressure will build. This pressure represents energies which we absorb which can under healthy circumstances be repelled, bounced off, released, or diminished. The energy that we absorb has to go somewhere. We all are familiar with a rubber band absorbing energy as it is stretched. When it is released, it resumes its original state with the release of the absorbed energy. Similarly, our muscles and ligaments readily absorb energy and when they do, they contract to become shorter, stiffer, and tighter, and this process is typically accompanied by increasing pain. The muscles which are commonly affected are the heart and stomach which are essentially large muscles, as well as all the muscles and ligaments of our musculoskeletal system.

Just as an initial overload of pressure in the tea kettle might be thought of as causing pain at the weakest link, or links, or even the entire kettle in some cases, absorption of excess stress energy can initially give a warning pain signal kind of like a warning signal on the car dashboard. This warning signal generally is not yet urgent or an emergency, however, must be heeded. The appropriate reaction is first to notice and be aware of the signal, then to stop everything, take a time out, whether it's with your car or your body, figure out what the problem and source of the problem is, and make appropriate fixes, changes, or corrections.

If this warning signal is not heeded, then what was initially a buildup of pressure in the tea kettle can turn into a rupture of the body of the kettle. Similarly, an overload of stress energy in a muscle, body part, collection of muscles or body parts, or even the entire body, initially presents as pain. This pain can turn into "an explosion" such as a heart attack, ruptured ulcer of the stomach, cancer, or any type of muscle, tendon, ligament, or joint rupture, tear, or herniation.

The tea kettle model demonstrates a fine balance of processes. First is the fire burning, next is the kettle containing and constraining the water and steam, then the water transforms to steam, and next the kettle spout accommodates the release of energy from the system. We humans must exhibit the same delicate balance of processes if we are to maintain our health and wholeness and avoid diseases of all types.

More:

Once upon a time a poor old lady was forced to sell her valuables to avoid eviction. As she rummaged through her dusty belongings, she came across a dull copper kettle. Intrigued by its possible value the old woman dusted it off and suddenly a genie appeared. The genie said, "I know of your struggles and will grant you three wishes." The woman was astounded, thought for a moment, and said, "Age has taken its toll on me. I wish to be young and beautiful once more."

No sooner had she spoken than she turned into a beautiful young woman. Thrilled by her success she said, "Genie, I want to be rich!" With a snap of the genie's fingers the room transformed into a great hall and her once broken-down cottage became a mansion. She noticed that her worn clothing had been replaced with a beautiful stunning dress and shoes.

The genie then said to her, "You have one wish left." The woman thought for a while and then felt her cat brush against her leg. Her cat had been with her forever. The woman turned to the genie and said, "This cat has remained faithful to me for all my years. Please transform him into a handsome man so that we may spend the rest of our lives together!"

The cat vanished immediately. Standing in its place was a tall handsome young man, and the woman fell directly into his arms. The genie's work was done, so he disappeared. As the woman gazed into her new love's eyes, he drew her close and whispered, "Too bad you had me neutered."

This story is relevant because the woman was old, alone, and soon to be evicted. Clearly, she had her challenges. The tea kettle model offers practical real-life analysis and help for such problems. The path to recovery requires a positive attitude and action to make helpful change. The tea kettle provides us with a useful analogy and is not a magical tool. The kettle in this story, however, is magical. Wishful thinking and hoping for magical answers in life can never substitute for taking action.

17

Lobster Medicine

U nderstanding and experiencing happiness and joy can give great peace and balance to one's life. One's mental attitude, mental outlook, and mental health can be determined by their ability to experience happiness and joy. Different people have different life experiences making the journey to understanding and living with happiness and joy a very personal one. We have so many obstacles and challenges in life that it is hard not to feel tied up. Sometimes we are immediately successful in an endeavor, but very often, we struggle over and over with life challenges and overcoming barriers. When we don't succeed, it is effortless to become sad and depressed. We can even give up and escaping through addiction or suicide is a common outcome.

We all experience the greatest repetitive failure in our lives as infants. The process of advancing from crawling to standing is a long, drawn-out process consisting of many repetitive failed attempts to stand. No child determines that they'll never be successful and gives up, and neither does any parent give up on their child labeling them a failure. Later in life, whether during young years of schooling or during adulthood, many people consider themselves failures in various endeavors and undertakings in life. But we know that very often what distinguishes one who is successful from one who is not is his fortitude in overcoming temporary "failure" and never giving up.

The successful person has self-esteem and self-confidence and doesn't let a temporary "fall" in the ongoing attempt and struggle to stand get them down or discourage them. They maintain a positive attitude, pick themselves up and brush themselves off after any fall, and push on towards their goal. The individual falls or failings are only failings if you let them be. They can equally well be tremendous learning experiences and practice in the process of gaining the wisdom and know-how to finally achieve success. It's all according to one's attitude and whether you can have the attitude, approach, drive, and joy of the infant and its parents. The infant's falls on its journey from a crawler to a walker are never failures, and your "falls" in life should not be considered failures either.

The process of battling on with strength and courage through struggles and challenges in life in the process of breaking through so many of the barriers that tie us up and restrict us is a never-ending one. Just as the infant that conquers the ability to stand transforms from the identity of a crawler to the elevated identity of a walker, every time we break a barrier, we, too, undergo an elevating transformation. This process is repeated over and over in our lifetime. Despite a massive change in who we are because of this barrier-breaking process of transformation, there is typically no concomitant visible outward change in our appearance.

We begin our lives as babies, little people, and as we grow older into adulthood and beyond, we become bigger, but basically, we are recognizable as the same person and creation. When we encounter and engage challenges and obstacles, the process does not typically produce any outward visible transformative change, yet often an internal change does occur. To better understand what is really happening through this change, it helps to examine the life cycle of two different creatures that also undergo transformative change, albeit a different type.

First is the butterfly. The butterfly starts as a caterpillar. The caterpillar does lots of eating and growing. At a certain point, the caterpillar creates a cocoon for itself within which it disappears. The cocoon is a place of hiding and separation from the outside world. It is a barrier formed by the caterpillar, creating a place of darkness, silence, and vulnerability. While in the cocoon, significant transformative physical change occurs, and when the time is right, the creature emerges as a beautiful winged flying butterfly. This transformative metamorphosis occurs a single time in the lifecycle of the butterfly.

Next is the lobster. The lobster is a soft creature that has a hard outer shell. The inner soft animal continually grows throughout its life while the hard-exoskeletal shell is fixed in size and is not compliant. The lobster grows increasing in size until the outer shell becomes confining and painful, no longer accommodating the size of the lobster. The lobster then finds an isolated hidden dark crevice to escape to and in that space sheds its shell. Without its protective shell, the soft creature is then totally vulnerable as food for any other creatures. Once out of its shell, it imbibes a lot of water and grows even bigger before it creates a new comfortable shell. Once it is protected in its new shell, it leaves its hiding place. The lifecycle of the lobster involves repeated episodes of molting or shedding of its confining shell and creating a new, larger, more accommodating shell. This process, which occurs many times in the life of the lobster, has similarities singular caterpillar to butterfly transformation.

Both the lifecycle of the butterfly and the lobster share a monumental transformative visible physical metamorphosis. These transformations are both characterized by a period of separation, darkness, quiet, and vulnerability. This process of physical change is not a choice for these creatures, but instead is a pre-programmed part of their lives as ordained by the Creator. The change for both creatures is about the formation of an advanced, new and improved version of themselves.

These transformative changes in the life of the butterfly and lobster serve as wonderful models for the many changes which occur in the lives of human beings. Our Divine Soul can be compared to the soft lobster creature. As we feed our Divine Soul with faith, learning G0dly wisdom, prayer, and performing acts of lovingkindness, the Divine Soul grows. The

Divine Soul is confined by the physical human body and by restrictive thoughts, speech, and action imposed by the outside world. Often many times in the human life cycle, we go through a process of transformative metamorphosis not unlike that of the caterpillar to butterfly transformation and the molting of the lobster. The difference is that whereas for the butterfly and lobster, it is a physical transformation, for humans, it is not a physical transformation, but instead is a Soul or Spiritual transformation.

We are all familiar with the "terrible twos," the teenage years of rebellion, "midlife crises," and personal life stories of encountering and dealing with many different types of life struggles and challenges. What all of these battles share is a desire of the Soul to overcome and conquer a "tied-up," restrictive, confining, painful "Shell" like that of the lobster. There are many sources of this confining shell including a variety of afflictions. Addiction to eating, cigarettes, alcohol, or drugs is one group of sources. Disease and injury are another group of sources. A partial list includes obesity, low back pain and other muscle and joint pains, heart disease, hypertension, diabetes, cancer, depression, Parkinson's disease, multiple sclerosis, cerebral palsy, muscular dystrophy, amputation, cancer, and any other physical challenge of the body or from outside the body. This shell can also be an externally imposed or internally created thought, speech, or action and involve relationships of all types as well as social, work, and financial interactions.

The Divine Soul's process of breaking free from confining constraining shells can be purposely and consciously motivated, or it can be driven by a deep-seated unconscious hunger of the Divine Soul for freedom and "fresh air." The Soul transformation we experience as a result of this process can be as stark and drastic as the physical transformation of the butterfly and lobster. With each change, we overcome a barrier to reaching higher spiritual heights, and our Divine Soul becomes stronger, larger, and more connected and closer to G0d.

This process in humans can be very deceptive because as monumental as the transformative metamorphosis is, it is a nonphysical Soul Transformation. There may be associated physical changes such as healthy modification of eating habits, stopping of smoking, drinking, or drugs, visible change in use of the mouth to speak and eat, and other changes. However, these outward visible changes are minuscule compared to the real change which is nonphysical invisible Soul change. This nonphysical Soul change is as dramatic as the transformative physical change of the butterfly and lobster.

The transformation of crawling multi-legged caterpillar to a beautiful multi-colored winged flying butterfly is a wonderful model to understand how amazingly beautiful the human Soul Transformation can be and how the human Divine Soul can soar like the butterfly. This model is limited though, in that the caterpillar transforms into a butterfly only once in its lifetime. The lobster model is also a wonderful model to explain the human transformative experience. The lobster model demonstrates the process of breaking free from the painful confining constrictive shell, a process similar to what we experience as humans. Unlike the butterfly, lobsters undergo this transformation multiple times in their lives.

Similar to the lobster lifecycle, we experience the process of Soul Transformation multiple times in our lifetimes. There is always some kind of barrier, challenge, or struggle to tackle and overcome. Once we succeed in overcoming one barrier, it is easy to think we have arrived, and the challenges are over. But they are never over. After completing each Soul Transformation, although the Divine Soul is at a higher level, and there is a great sense of accomplishment, a whole new challenge and associated transformation will present. This process repeats throughout our lifetime as it does for the lobster.

Worthy of discussion is how the caterpillar and lobster both retreat to an isolated separated space characterized by darkness and silence. Very often to hear ourselves think, to block external distractions, diversions, and deception and to create a comfortable space to transform, we need our own safe space offering silence, darkness, and separateness just like the caterpillar and lobster. We can choose to undergo healthy transformative Soul change. Yet, sometimes without conscious choice or even having the slightest bit of understanding about what is happening, we find ourselves in a place of darkness, silence, separation, and vulnerability. This process can be smooth, controlled, and even seamless with little to no pain. It also can be harrowing, frightening, very lonely, and very painful.

More:

Franz Kafka's "The Metamorphosis" was about the life of a young man who on awakening one morning found himself transformed into a cockroach. Suddenly his new body seemed to represent all the pains and sorrows of his life. He did not care for his job as a traveling salesman and cloth merchant. He did not like his employer or the office manager. He was unhappy as his family's sole breadwinner straddled with the job of working off his bankrupt father's debts. His new cockroach body might symbolize the enormous paralyzing weight of his life struggles.

In the case of "The Metamorphosis", a horrific physical transformation takes place symbolizing the struggles of our existence. The antidote to feeling boxed in is a Soul Transformation that enables a shedding of confining restrictions. This human metamorphosis is well worth understanding and experiencing. It is an invisible change whereby the Soul sheds its confining shell like the lobster, and gains wings of freedom and liberation like that of the butterfly.

18

Depression, Manic Depression, Schizophrenia and Your Mental Health

W e have been talking about a new paradigm for understanding obesity and addiction based on identity not of the body but the nonphysical Divine Soul. Since the Soul must work through the physical body to actualize its desires, a well-functioning healthy body is essential. The chief machine through which the Soul uses the body is the brain. If the brain is compromised in some way, such as with a mental illness, then the ability to live a fulfilled life as one's Soul identity is challenged. The medical profession as a whole, including the specialties of psychiatry and psychology, generally negates the concepts of G0d and Soul, making our new paradigm untenable in the healthcare system as it currently exists.

The medical profession also readily creates stigmatized disease labels for all kinds of behaviors and conditions, which are generally attributed to some combination of genetics, environment, bodily produced chemicals, injury, and other causes. The incidence of the combined conditions of depression, manic depression, and schizophrenia is very high affecting many people. These are disease labels with lifelong stigmas from the perspective of both the patient and the public. Perhaps from the perspective of our new paradigm, there might be a different way of understanding what is happening with these patients, and a different pathway to achieving good health.

Depression has been attributed to genetics, chemical imbalance, and situational circumstances. It is considered by almost everyone including professionals and the public to be an abnormal disease state. It is treated with anti-depression medication, counseling, electric shock therapy, and other medical techniques. It has a high rate of occurrence in the general population, and no one is immune. All of this is based on the premise that we are a body with no Soul and no God. Once we allow the Divine Soul and G0d into our framework of thinking, new possibilities arise for understanding the conditions labeled as mental illness.

As anyone who has experienced depression knows, it is a state of disconnection from the outside world and often even from oneself. It typically comes on stealthily without warning. Thinking becomes foggy with a loss of ability to think clearly. Memory can become deficient. The senses of smell and taste are often dulled. Previous desires and interests wane. I believe that what we human beings are experiencing in this state is similar to the cocoon phase of the caterpillar and the molting phase of the lobster.

The process of physical transformation for the caterpillar and lobster is characterized by darkness, quiet, vulnerability, and separation. Human depression similarly seems to be a time of relative darkness, quiet, weakness, and separation. We discussed how Soul Transformation can be purposeful but may also be part of a subconsciously occurring process not under the direction of the individual. Perhaps what we human beings are experiencing during depression is a normal, natural process rather than a disease. Maybe depression is a sign of Soul Hunger and a need for G0dliness in one's life. It could be a process programmed into us, no different from that of the cocoon and molting stages in the lives of the caterpillar and lobster.

If this were the correct understanding of the meaning of depression, then it would be a normal, natural process rather than a disease. If this were common knowledge and depression did not have a bad stigma, then the pathway out of this phase of "darkness, silence, vulnerability, and separation" would be by satisfying the underlying Soul Hunger with Soul Food. Learning to find and establish one's true identity as the Divine Soul and seeking closeness and connection with G0d by growing one's faith, learning, thinking, and speaking G0dly wisdom, praying, and performing acts of lovingkindness are all nourishment for the Soul. Strengthening one's healthy relationships and connections and abandoning unhealthy ones are also essential. Further help to facilitate a healthy productive Soul Transformation derives from knowing that everything comes from G0d and therefore is for the good, and that the phase of depression is temporary. Other valuable therapeutic tools are keeping a positive attitude, making or listening to soothing, joyful music, and doing healthy exercise.

What is being facilitated is the elevation and growth of the Divine Soul from the "cocoon phase" consisting of darkness, silence, vulnerability, and separation to the wonderful and beautiful "butterfly phase." The Divine Soul is wanting to throw off its shackles and become so much freer like the lobster shedding its shell. Unlike the caterpillar and lobster which undergo their physical transformations instinctually and seamlessly, we humans often need other humans to help us in many circumstances, and especially in times of pain, trouble, and confusion. Kind, warm, and understanding facilitators to help those of us undergoing Soul Transformation, both individually and in groups, via guided connection to our Divine Soul identity and to G0d, might very possibly be a tremendous help to the global state of mental health.

With the current paradigm of understanding and treatment of depression, it becomes a self-fulfilling state of being. The depressed individual, their family, friends, and acquaintances, and their healthcare providers all assume that genetics or chemical imbalances are the cause of the depression and that a depressed behavior with a negative attitude and negative thoughts is to be expected. There is no understanding or acceptance of the concepts of or existence of the Soul or G0d. With no notion of the Soul, there can be no concept of Soul Food or Soul Hunger.

Furthermore, if genetics or a chemical imbalance is the cause, how in the world can anyone or any doctor overcome this strong programming from the body? Perhaps genetics has nothing to do with depression other than it possibly occurs as a learned behavior from a parent or other family member or close person. Many familial behaviors may not be of a genetic nature but may instead be passed on by "psychological genetics" as learned behaviors.

Regarding the explanation that depression is caused by a chemical imbalance, this is but a theory and seems flawed. The question boils down to the old paradox of which came first, the chicken or the egg. Does a change in bodily chemicals cause a change in behavior, thinking, and attitude, or does a change in behavior, thinking, and attitude cause a change in chemicals? Thinking of depression as a disease state, it makes sense to believe that genetics or a brain and body chemical imbalance are the cause.

Another possibility is that depression is not a disease state and instead is a normal healthy human process of Soul growth. Underlying this transformation might be a change of brain function to question the previous "normal" order of things and cause doubt, confusion, lack of self-confidence, negative thinking, and a sense of emptiness. The impetus for this change might be a natural desire to fill the void of a lack of knowledge of oneself as a Divine Soul and lack of understanding and connection to G0d. In this paradigm, habitually thinking motivated positive thoughts would produce "positive behavior chemicals" and habitually thinking negative thoughts would produce "negative behavior chemicals."

In the new paradigm we have a toolbox of powerful instruments for healing. Positive thinking knowing that since everything is from G0d it is all for the good, having faith and trust in G0d even when things don't seem good, and learning to connect with oneself as Divine Soul and with G0d are one set of tools. It is also essential to recognize that depression is a temporary transitional state in the process of Soul Transformation to become a beautiful butterfly. All of these tools and perhaps changing the name from the very stigmatized "depression" to a new more palatable and more positive term, like PB for Pre-Butterfly (or peanut butter), might be helpful to cheer up many suffering people and shed some light on what is currently a very dark behavioral malady.

Manic depression or bipolar disorder is very different from depression, and here again, we are told that it is a behavior caused by genetics or chemical imbalances in the body. As with depression, medicine looks at this behavior as a purely bodily process with no consideration that Soul or G0d may play a role because, according to medical science, they do not exist. Yet bipolar disorder is easily explained once Soul and G0d are acknowledged as real. First, it is helpful to recognize that a wave form that waxes and wanes with ups and downs, peaks and troughs, or highs and lows is commonplace in nature.

Sound waves, light waves, the waves of the ocean, and the pattern of sunlight during day and night all exhibit a pattern of change consisting of peaks and troughs. A similar pattern can be found in our brain waves, heart rhythm, speech, and breathing, as well as the daily pattern of cycling between being awake and asleep. We are not static creatures and instead are part of nature, so highs and lows are built into our natural makeup as well. If we naturally live as a wave form, is there a way to optimize our balance and avoid extreme problematic highs and lows?

We have previously discussed how the Divine Soul is not whole and is incomplete by itself. We human beings and our Divine Soul get our identity by completing ourselves by connecting with people, places, and things outside of our Divine Soul. Choosing and prioritizing these connections wisely will determine one's degree of wholeness, peace, and balance. Since our bodies are temporary and in fact everything we can connect to except G0d is temporary, the number one connection a human being can make to achieve true wholeness and balance is with G0d.

Only G0d always was, always is, and always will be. Making connections with anything else but G0d will tend to allow extreme behavioral variances in one's life, especially if you are driven by passion. For example, today, working out to have a strong body causes a high. Then you sprain your ankle and you get low. Then you get high on a girlfriend. Then she breaks up with you and you get low. Then you get high on a rising stock market. Then the market crashes and you get low.

This type of identity dependence on changing things external to the Soul, without stability and balance promoted by connection to G0d, the unwavering Rock, can seem like a mental disease caused by genetics or chemical imbalances. But that is only if G0d and Soul do not exist and are not brought into the equation of understanding and unraveling such common human behavior. As with depression, "psychological genetics" may play a role in determining behavior. But regarding chemical imbalances, it makes little sense that chemical changes suddenly occur and cause behavioral changes. Much more feasible is that mental attitude and passions producing highs and lows are the cause of chemical changes.

A positive or elevated attitude would cause the production of chemicals that promote a positive or elevating attitude, and a negative or depressed attitude would cause production of chemicals that promote a negative or depressed attitude. Once we understand the role our Soul and G0d play in our behavior, the behavior labeled as manic depression or bipolar disease becomes a normal process of life. The solution then becomes helping and facilitating the affected individual to find their new identity as the Divine Soul and helping them to build a strong primary connection to G0d. Focusing one's passion primarily toward G0d rather than toward other things will lead to understanding, calm, peace, and balance.

Schizophrenia means a "split mind" and is the term for a reality disorder. We previously encountered this word when considering the two conflicting personalities of the human being, the Divine Soul and the Animal Soul. A schism and inability to find a balance between these two souls can present as one form of schizophrenia.

Schizophrenia is known to occur in very intelligent people. We can imagine people who subconsciously are disturbed by the fact that the world of human interaction is full of deception, distraction, and diversion. This subconscious awareness can be excruciating, especially to a brilliant and sensitive Soul. To combat this awareness and pain, as a healthy survival mechanism, the person can subconsciously gradually create a false imaginary world for themselves to dull the pain. They are not part of a religious community that purposely resides in two worlds with harmony, so as they build their imaginary protective world apart from any community and anyone else, they become more and more isolated.

Living as the Divine Soul, connecting with G0d, and being part of a supportive community might well be the antidote for this behavior. The sooner this behavior is realized, and alignment with the solution is offered, the higher the chance of a healthy outcome. The longer one goes, and the deeper one becomes in their isolated way of thinking, the less the chance they will do well. Here again, "psychological genetics" can play a role, and chemical changes would tend to follow changes in thought processes rather than vice versa. Hope for a healthy outcome is offered by early facilitation, especially in a group setting, but also individually to identify as the Divine Soul and connect with G0d to bring understanding to these affected individuals.

It is possible that the mental health state of America could be vastly improved by changing our approach and attitude toward and treatment of these behaviors, including depression, bipolar disorder, and schizophrenia. The new paradigm and treatment "diet" for these conditions, which are currently treated as mental health diseases involves removing the currently used stigmatized labels and creating facilitators for individuals and, most importantly, groups as well. A large number of people struggle and suffer from mental instability. The importance of teaching and advancing the new paradigm in groups is about reinforcement. The current mode of understanding and treatment, which by the way has mainly been unsuccessful, will be what many people including healthcare providers, family, friends, and community will try to implement on those seeking help. Daily moment by moment positive reinforcement is crucial. This pathway could lead to considerable improvement in health, a huge cost saving, and decreased need for doctor visits, hospitalization, medication, and treatments of all kinds.

More:

In the times before modern technology, water was not readily available in homes, and it was up to the local water carrier to deliver water to each home. The water carrier would use a harness that ran over his upper back and to each shoulder and from each of which hung a large pot filled with water. One water carrier had been delivering water to his community for many years and he knew that one of his pots had a small crack in it. One day after his deliveries, he was surprised to hear his cracked pot apologize to him for having a crack and for leaking water and for not being able to do the same job as the other pot.

He then immediately took his pots on a walk to show them how he felt about the cracked pot and what it had said. They took a long walk visiting all the areas they had walked along over the years. He pointed out to the cracked pot that where it had passed and leaked water beautiful plants and flowers grew, yet where the intact pot had passed, there were no plants or flowers.

The moral of this story is that we all have unique flaws making each one of us a cracked pot. The singer, songwriter, and poet, Leonard Cohen is known for singing, "There is a crack in everything. That's how the light gets in." It's not so bad to be a crackpot. Even for a crackpot, beautiful things are possible. It is important to be kind, forgiving, and appreciative of ourselves and other people.

19

The Therapeutic Power of Crying and Laughter

L obster medicine explains how our internal soft essential aspect is the nonphysical growing Divine Soul that has the holy desire to serve G0d selflessly. This essence is encased in a hard-outer exoskeletal shell that is motivated by the Animal Soul. It consists of our body and those thoughts, speech, and actions which have separated us from G0d. Soul growth of the human being depends on multiple Soul Transformations, a process that resembles the physical transformations which are essential to the lives of the butterfly and the lobster.

The process of Soul Transformation is complex and often is accompanied by pain and monumental struggle. But there are times in our lives when we experience mini Soul Transformations and windows to understanding this most complex process. These are times when we are touched and moved by internal thought and revelation or by external stimuli to cry or laugh. Our normal state of existence is our soft Divine Soul essence enclosed our hard exterior. This hard exterior can be likened to the shell of a walnut which must be cracked to reach the fruit it contains. Soul Transformation to allow Soul growth requires a "cracking of the walnut shell." This process is also like that of a chicken hatching from its egg.

Sensitivity to pain or joy can lead to crying and a momentary cracking of the walnut shell from the inside out. Crying connects one with some profound truth and momentarily all of the confining outer layers of lies and deception that have created separation from G0d melt away. Similarly, laughter is typically brought on by hearing or seeing something truthful that is rarely expressed, or that is shown in an unusual way that causes a sudden shift in one's perception of reality. Laughter is a momentary "cracking of the walnut" from the outside in. Both crying and laughter can affect the body so profoundly that a rippling effect is experienced. This rippling effect is analogous to the cracking of the walnut and is a temporary experience of shedding one's shell like the molting of the lobster.

This transformative cleansing effect is why crying and laughter are both known to be therapeutic and sometimes are described as "the best medicine." They both offer a temporary sense of freedom from all that ties us up and from pain. They both create an out of body experience where the Divine Soul essence is manifested and is palpably felt. Pursuit of this state of being is a worthwhile goal. Claiming our identity as Divine Soul and connecting with G0d help forge the necessary path.

More:

Bringing laughter to others is a noble calling, especially when people are struggling and filled with pain and sadness. Comedy used to be innocent and was about exposing the foibles of human nature. Comedians typically are born of their own personal experience of pain or of a sensitivity to all the pain around them. Even if for only a brief time, the classical comedians of yesterday were in the business of removing our pain and giving us an innocent pleasurable out of body experience.

The proof of the purity of the old humor was that it was for everyone.

It was not offensive to anyone. Today comedians use foul language and attack politics and politicians, religion, race, ethnicity, etc. Much of what is offered up as comedy today is offensive to many and has lost the beautiful human touch of the comedy of old. Nothing compares to watching the old-time comedians on social media and having a good hearty laugh.

20

The MD, MRI, Meds, and Surgery Windmill-Navigating the Healthcare Maze

It seems that everyone has health problems at one time or another, and no matter who you are or what lifestyle you choose to lead, the years of your life are limited, and no one gets out of here alive. We have seen how one's identity and freedom are determined by their choice of diet paradigm. Choosing a bodily identity or that of the Animal Soul ties you up or imprisons you in many forms of servitude to a multitude of false gods. Choosing the identity of the Divine Soul gives you the ultimate freedom of servitude to G0d.

We as Divine Souls are trapped in our bodies including when we are in good health. Despite the ability and necessity to utilize our bodies to accomplish our divine purpose and mission, we are restricted by the body's physical limitations. How much more so when our health is challenged?

The freedom of the Divine Soul to accomplish its mission is diminished when the body experiences health problems.

It is so vital to maintain one's identity as Divine Soul with the ultimate mission of connecting with and selflessly serving G0d, both in good health and in times of poor health. The medical profession and healthcare do not generally acknowledge the existence of Soul or G0d. When G0d-the Creator of all, the Source of everything, the ultimate and only Healer, and the Rock-is not recognized, that is when a potentially infinite number of false gods are created and empowered by man. There is probably nowhere that this is more apparent than in healthcare.

Physical illness is a time of compromise. Energy and strength are limited, yet optimal personal strength and power are vitally necessary to combat, conquer, and recover from any disease. It would be desirable to be able to muster more energy and strength than one normally possesses to be able to combat the extra burden of disease. Many people don't just get medical advice and treatment, but instead surrender their willpower and strength. The healthcare system, its doctors and healthcare providers, hospitals, medications, tests, procedures, X-rays, MRI's, and surgeries are often granted ultimate power. Consequently, from the patient's perspective, any of these components of the healthcare system can usurp the role of G0d.

The public generally is not learned in physical disease processes and pathways of healing. This lack of knowledge and understanding mandates that we seek help from the healthcare system. Medical practice is based on the knowledge and treatment of the human being as a body with organ systems and body parts that experience a variety of disease states. For the most part, this practice works exclusive of concepts of Soul and G0d. Based on our diet paradigm, this seems to be a paradox worth exploring.

For a healthy individual whose identity is their Divine Soul connected to G0d, health and healing is all about the Soul directing the function of the body in conjunction with healing energy and power provided by G0d directly to the body. In a disease state, reevaluating and strengthening the Soul's management of the body, and seeking more healing energy from

G0d is desirable. However, once the healthcare system is entered, healing is promoted often without acknowledging the Soul and G0d and their incredible significance to health and healing. In a system where Soul and God are absent, by default, the doctor and hospital, medications, tests, X-rays, MRI's, procedures, and surgeries assume the role of god and healer.

As human beings, G0d has endowed us with two processes that are present within us throughout our lives. These are aging and healing. Every cell, organ, and body part are always aging and healing. We become familiar with healing at a young age when we first scrape our skin. Mom cleans you off and applies a band-aid to the scrape to hide it from your vision. Over time the scrape heals and disappears. By the time we are adults, a scrape is not a concern, yet it can take several months for a scrape to heal and the skin to remodel. Although scientists can describe the healing process, they have no idea how it is orchestrated, how the body knows what to do, or how to reproduce it. We don't have to tell our brain to focus twenty-four hours a day on making the skin heal. As long as we don't abuse our bodies and reinjure the area, the skin heals seamlessly in spite of us.

This process of healing of the body is a combination of the Divine Soul's careful use of the body and absorption of healing energy from G0d. The body is the intermediate between and is acted on by both the Soul and G0d. In our diet paradigm, it is essential to recognize the important, influential roles that the Divine Soul and G0d play in bodily healing. Contrary to one form of prevalent thinking, the body does not heal itself.

Our relationship with G0d in healing is similar to the process of photosynthesis in plants. The Soul derives its life force from G0d. Just as we need G0d's light to survive, all plants need sunlight for growth. What if well-intentioned scientists wanted to increase the sunlight reaching a plant and made a magnifying glass to do so? They would burn and kill the plant. What if they created a stronger device in the form of a laser? They would burn and kill the plant even faster. A clear prism or pane of glass that allows the sunlight to pass through will allow the plant to thrive. An opaque prism that completely blocks light passage will eventually kill the plant.

Similar to the hypothetical use of technology to modify the delivery of sunlight to plants, doctors are trained to come at us with technologies and surgeries to promote healing. Some methods have good results while others are not successful. Doctors and their tools can usurp the healing roles of Divine Soul and God, either because they genuinely feel a need to do something or because of a profit motive. Nonetheless, often the best treatment would be the "clear pane of glass" or "Do no harm" approach that simply promotes healing from the Divine Soul and G0d without any advanced technologies.

We know "Do no harm" as the Hippocratic oath and credo. Many doctors assume, with all good intentions and based on their training, that their skills are necessary for healing. They are often oblivious to the Soul and God and how they both endow the body with healing power. Therefore, it is common for doctors to assume that if they don't act, healing will not occur.

Primary care doctors are trained to take measurements, make corresponding diagnoses, and prescribe medication. If a patient has pain of any sort, the primary care physician has limited resources and knowledge. They can prescribe Tylenol, aspirin, Motrin, Naprosyn, or other medication, but if the pain persists for one to two weeks or whatever the doctor's threshold of tolerance for the patient's pain is, they will then refer the patient to a specialist.

Often by obtaining an MRI study, which generally results in a report of some kind of a clinical diagnosis, the primary care physician can validate referral of the patient to the specialist. The specialist generally won't see the patient unless there is reason to believe that surgery will be a treatment option. The specialist, like the primary care physician, also has a threshold of tolerance for the patient's pain, and generally once it is met, surgery will be recommended. Many pain conditions such as low back pain can take up to three, six, or even twelve months for pain resolution and healing. However, the patient wants immediate relief, and because the specialist doesn't want to listen to the patient complain over more than perhaps two or three visits, surgery may be performed before adequate time for healing has occurred.

Non-recognition of the role of G0d and Soul in healing, and concomitant lack of understanding of how we are made and how long healing takes are common. Subsequently, doctors and patients often push for surgeries well before healing has been given enough time to occur. These unnecessary and inappropriate surgeries will allow the patient time off to recover and a lengthy course of physical therapy, with no guaranteed result. If the patient had taken time off and undergone physical therapy without surgery, in time they may have experienced a better result than with surgery. Doctors and patients are both driven by the "quick fix push-button" mentality. Many doctors have come to see themselves and their treatments as gods and are motivated to administer a "quick fix" to the patients. Likewise, many patients see the doctors and their treatments as gods and desire a "quick fix." They are both experiencing a temporary state of insanity, even if the doctor might be sanely motivated by a profit motive.

Whereas the goal of healthcare should be to restore health, wellness, happiness, and wholeness to the patient, there is a silent rarely recognized opposite force lurking in the healthcare system. The word doctor is from the Latin word docere, meaning teacher. Doctor does not mean surgerizer or pillerizer. It means to elevate the patient and help make them whole, to "do no harm," and to "not put a stumbling block before the blind."

The process of educating and making a doctor, however, is often a process of taking a whole person and gradually whittling away at their humanity. The education of a doctor progresses from youthful open-mindedness, to focusing on a single subject in college, to identifying with a single profession in medical school, to working in a unique specialty or subspecialty in training. They become a hammer hungry to hit a nail. They are trained to have a "shark" mentality and are driven by the profit motive to apply their new identity and tools to anyone and everyone.

Doctors are reported to have the highest degree of unhappiness, divorce, drug addiction, and suicide of all professions, and this can be attributed to this painful process of the sacrifice of their wholeness. They are also a victim of an underlying psychological force that drives them to do to their patients what has been done to them. Instead of helping patients in need connect with their true identities as Divine Souls and with G0d, they exert a similar "whittling down" process on the patients as was applied to themselves. They turn the patient from a whole human being into a diseased body part and a medical label and they make the patient the nail to their hammer. This process is a painful one for the patient.

The typical patient is confronting a disease process that is coming from inside themselves and which they cannot see. Since their attacker is from within and they cannot see it, they are unable to mount an adequate defense. They typically see the doctor as their helper and think the doctor loves them, and often make them into all-knowing and all-powerful gods. All the while, the doctor is actually attacking them by shrinking their identity and doing the opposite of delivering wholeness, and by prescribing pills and doing surgery. The patient finally has a "friendly" outside attacker that they can see and mount a defense to and eventually heal. This process of healing and becoming whole is despite the doctor and his intention.

An additional powerful force helping to drive a large volume of surgeries for profit motive is the MRI. MRI is one of the most worshipped gods of the current day and the way it is utilized plays a huge role in defying our diet paradigm. A bit of history is necessary to understand what is meant by this. In 1971-72 nuclear magnetic resonance (NMR) was found to be able to distinguish between healthy human tissue and cancer tissue. In 1974 Dr. Damadian a physician at Downstate Medical Center in Brooklyn, NY, received several patents towards making the first magnetic resonance imaging (MRI) machine to detect cancer. He did not call it NMRI for fear of frightening people with the word "nuclear." In 1977 he made the first MRI machine at Downstate Medical Center and used it to make the first MRI images on a coworker. He did so for the noble purpose of being able to detect cancer.

Profit motive immediately reared its head and a large number of wealthy companies including General Electric, Phillips, Siemens, and others violated Dr. Damadian's patents and began making copies of his MRI invention. Soon in the early 1980s, a handful of MRI machines appeared in several major medical centers for the sole purpose of detecting cancer.

Within the first several years of use, MRI was found to be equally valuable for detecting infection. From the beginning of its use, MRI images were interpreted by radiologists reading the images in a back room never seeing the patients and never performing a patient history or physical examination. It was a lackluster job.

Then the radiologists became glorified when they surreptitiously added new functionality to the MRI. When they were looking at images of the head for cancer or infection, they also saw the cervical spine. When they were looking at the chest, they also saw the shoulders and thoracic spine. When they were looking at the pelvis, they also saw the lumbosacral spine and hips. They began reporting on incidental findings unrelated to cancer or infection such as cervical and lumbosacral disc herniation, rotator cuff tear of the shoulder, and torn meniscus of the knee. These are clinical diagnoses and cannot be determined from MRI images alone. These diagnoses can only be adequately made after obtaining a proper medical history and physical examination of the patient.

The radiologists could have simply described what they saw on the MRI images. Such descriptions might have included: the C5-6 disk extends 3 mm posterior to the posterior longitudinal ligament, or there is a linear lucency in the supraspinatus tendon of the right shoulder, or there is a linear lucency in the posterior horn of the medial meniscus. These descriptions are non-threatening for patients compared to the words "herniation" and "tear" which suggest the patient is "damaged" and that this is the source of the patient's pain. The radiologists' introduction of all these new diagnoses emanating from the use of MRI resulted in massive new business growth. The manufacture of MRI machines, the purchase and ownership of MRI machines by anyone and everyone with enough money including hospitals, surgery centers, doctors of all types, lawyers, business people, and others, their location anywhere including even strip malls, the utilization of MRI, and the generation of surgery based on MRI results have all experienced exponential skyrocketing growth.

Although the invention and inception of MRI was marked by noble intention, profit motive took over and the MRI became a god. Around the same time MRI was invented, Star Trek was a popular television show. On the show Dr. McCoy used a hand-held science fiction tool to diagnose and heal disease called the Tricorder device. This device was truly miraculous in its capability. From this science fiction creation, it was not difficult to see how this popular tv show and the device could impact the imagination of people, including doctors and patients, to believe that the MRI device had similar powers. MRI is a complex scientific concept and device. Yet many people, including doctors and patients, envision it as a magical god-like truth machine and believe that any report generated using MRI is the gospel. Going into the "black box" of the MRI machine will generate the answer to whatever your medical problem might be.

Unfortunately, this is far from the truth and those in the business of MRI, as well as doctors and patients, have all promoted the MRI as a self-fulfilling fantasy with massive profit motive. In fact, despite all the good, particularly for cancer and infection detection, the MRI can be likened to the Wizard of Oz or the Emperor with No Clothes. Several steps in the development and utilization of MRI have been and are totally flawed. These include the way MRI use was extended beyond cancer and infection detection, how the radiologists use clinical diagnostic labels rather than descriptions of what they see on MRI images to report MRI findings, and the assumption that whatever pain or problem a patient has is explained by the MRI report and findings.

A huge problem here is that this whole process often works against our diet paradigm. Our diet involves identifying as the Divine Soul and connecting with G0d and learning to live in the service of G0d. When pain strikes, it is essential to avoid anxiety, fear, depression, and anger. Any experience of pain is like a red light on the car dashboard. Cars are made with warning lights not to frighten anyone, but instead to give notification that action needs to be taken and can still be taken to avoid a significant problem. The car warning light is a signal to slow down or stop, evaluate the car and the overall situation, and address the situation so that it doesn't turn into a real problem or emergency.

Similarly, pain is a signal programmed by the Maker of our body, G0d, telling us to slow down or stop, avoid the use of the affected body part, evaluate the situation, and make appropriate changes. It is important to know that bodily healing is dependent on the Soul and G0d. The Godly Soul can be trained to promote bodily healing by thinking, speaking, and doing the right things, including avoiding abuse of affected body parts, eating healthy, doing meditative, focused, positive prayer and thinking, healthy bodily motion and exercise, and more.

Pain of the musculoskeletal system, which includes the muscles, tendons, bones, and joints, can be of three different sources. The most common cause of pain is related to the aging process and lifestyle. When we are young our body has a very high water content on a cellular and organic level. As we age, we lose water content. When we are young, our tissues are very fluid, and as we age, they become stiff, tight, and immobile. When we are young, we tend to have an active lifestyle compared to when we age and develop a sedentary lifestyle. As a result of these three processes acting over many years, muscles and ligaments shorten, stiffen, and tighten with age causing pain and stiffness.

The low back, neck, shoulders, and knees are most commonly affected, resulting in many doctor visits, MRIs, and surgeries. However, this most common source of pain is not detectable with MRI, so when MRIs are obtained for these patients, and incidental findings are found, they are often assumed to be the cause of the patient's pain, and unnecessary and inappropriate surgery is common. Generally, all that the patient would have required to achieve a good result would have been the avoidance of injury and overuse and a full range of motion program, time, and patience.

The next most common source of pain is of a nonphysical origin converting to a physical presentation of pain. This nonphysical source of pain comes from the Soul, intellect, and emotions, and includes a broken heart, pain related to failed endeavors, and all stressful occurrences and significant life changes such as a move, marriage, divorce, sickness, death, and other social, family, relationship, and financial troubles. Pain from any one of these or collection of these can readily translate into physical pain. This pain can occur anywhere and might be most likely to occur at the body's weakest link.

Weak links can result from physical deficiency, history of injury, or aging, or from psychologically derived weakness, such as having grown up with a parent who frequently complained about a specific body part. This second most common source of pain is not detectable with MRI. However, should MRI studies be obtained on these patients, there is a significant likelihood that surgery may be done, totally unrelated to the patient's source of pain.

The least common cause of musculoskeletal pain that patients might experience are the findings reported in MRI reports, including disc herniation of the neck and low back, rotator cuff tear of the shoulder, and torn meniscus of the knee. After an MRI is prescribed and obtained to help determine the cause of pain, the MRI report is transmitted to the patient. There is a high statistical chance that their pain is not from what is in the MRI report and instead is most likely from the first two most common causes explained above. is Unfortunately, this diagnostic dilemma is not common knowledge and is probably not explained enough to patients. Most patients are left with the understanding and assumption that their pain is a result of their MRI findings. It is not uncommon then for surgery to be planned based on a diagnosis that is not the cause of the patient's problem.

This drastic yet common dilemma is a by-product of a gigantic flaw that occurred in the development of MRI. MRI was initially developed as a miraculous tool to detect cancer and subsequently infection as well. When radiologists began reporting incidental findings as clinical diagnoses, they took this upon themselves without first questioning if this was a proper use of MRI and if what they were doing was truthful, safe, and not harmful. The fact that MRI was a perfect tool for the detection of cancer and infection should not have automatically translated into its use for a different purpose without first testing the validity of this application.

We have already seen how labeling with clinical diagnoses rather than descriptions of MRI image findings by radiologists is a misleading flaw in MRI utilization. These labels result in many unnecessary and inappropriate surgeries and, of course, are continued for a profit motive. Hospitals, surgical groups, doctors, radiologists, MRI owners, and MRI manufacturers all benefit in the pocketbook. If a radiologist were to do the right thing and report only image findings and not clinical diagnoses, they would probably lose their job.

But as problematic as all of this is, the flaw in MRI development and utilization is even more significant than that. Any time a new technology, test, or medication is created, before it can be used in humans, it needs to be adequately validated for safety. Statisticians must determine the statistically significant number of individuals needed to test validity and establish a baseline bell curve of normal findings. For MRI to be used to look for disc herniation, torn meniscus, and rotator cuff tear as diagnoses to explain patients' pain, first, we need to know what is "normal" in the general population. Establishing what normal is means selecting a statistically significant number of people in different age groupings for no history of pain or injury involving either the low back, neck, knee, or shoulder. The age groupings might by twenty to forty, forty to sixty, and sixty to eighty and above. It is crucially important to know what MRI images would reveal in these asymptomatic people. These results would allow for the determination of statistically significant baseline bell curve normal studies. These critical studies have never been done.

Currently the diagnoses coming from MRI reports are reported as "absolutes" as if the MRI machine is god and truth, the MRI report is god and truth, and the radiologist is god and truth. Results of other tests rarely never reported as absolutes and instead are reported as a range of normal values. Temperature, pulse, blood pressure, glucose, cholesterol, etc. are all reported as a value within a range of normal values. It was required of these tests and technologies that a statistically significant sampling of "normal" people was used to determine a bell curve and mean of normal values. This was never done with MRI.

The fifty-year-old woman with low back pain who is overweight and has a job, a husband, three children, and all the responsibilities of a homemaker, who is sent for an MRI of her low back is then called back the next week to speak with her primary care doctor. She is told that she has L4-5 disc herniation and may need surgery. A referral is made to the orthopedic surgeon. The word "herniation" is exceptionally frightening to her, and she assumes that she is "broken" and needs to be fixed. She is fearful and full of anxiety and doesn't know how she will handle surgery, work, or her family and home. This is all because of a word used by a radiologist who never met or evaluated the patient and is part of the routine process of radiologists never meeting or evaluating patients undergoing MRI studies, yet generating reports with fearful anxiety-producing diagnostic labels.

Statistically significant baseline bell curve normal studies have never been done. Therefore, crucial data that is necessary to use MRI results for decision-making is not available. Doctors who are savvy and care about their patients know experientially that roughly thirty percent of MRI's of healthy people by age thirty with no history of pain or injury would have findings of what radiologists call lumbar disc herniation, cervical disc herniation, torn meniscus of the knee, and rotator cuff tear of the shoulder. By age fifty, this finding goes up to about fifty percent, and by age seventy, it is approaching one hundred percent.

Many people receiving MRI studies are being frightened out of their minds by "herniation" and "tear" labels and are convinced that they are "broken" and that surgery is required. Many patients are oblivious that what they are being told is a significant problem is a normal finding for their age. Their pain and symptoms very often have absolutely nothing to do with the conclusions of the MRI report. There is a way to stop this gross injustice and harm to so many people perpetrated with MRI for profit motive. The use of MRI for evaluation of non-emergency low back, neck, knee, shoulder and other joint pain and problems should be halted until statistically significant baseline bell curve normal studies have been performed. While these studies are done the use of MRI for detecting cancer and infection can continue. Once the studies are completed, MRI study results can be reported more objectively, with less frightening labels, and with less propensity to drive surgery.

More:

During my first year of Jewish learning my dear uncle Joe passed on. I flew to Albany, New York where the funeral was held, and I attended Shabbos services with my relatives in the synagogue they belonged to. During the customary Torah reading, the reader stopped and was puzzled by a problem with the letters of one of the Hebrew words. That word is a verb referring to G0d putting Adam to sleep to create Eve. At this point, I was already questioning so much of what I had learned and experienced in medicine and was determined to unravel the truth. I took this problem with this particular word in the Torah as a personal sign of confirmation that G0d was not just the Creator of mankind and Adam's personal anesthesiologist and surgeon. G0d was in my eyes the ultimate and only true healer. Human doctors and their technologies can at most help or hinder a process of healing with G0d that is always ongoing.

The truth is that in all cases at all times, understanding of the science of G0dly healing and optimal promotion of this healing is essential. Doctors and the public would be helped by acknowledging that doctors are really in the business of facilitating G0dly healing. Proper lifestyle choices allowing the Soul to partner with G0d to induce a healthy effect on the body are always important. When medical technologies such as testing, medication, and surgery are utilized, care must always be taken to be sure G0dly healing is promoted rather than prevented. The right tool used in the right way at the right time in the right amount for the right patient can be miraculous. The same tool used improperly or at the wrong time or in the wrong amount or for the wrong patient can be deadly.

21

Taking a Surgical Vacation

Surgery means wielding a knife to address an anatomical problem. It's a process of bloodletting. In former times, various techniques of bloodletting, including knives and leeches, have been used. Bloodletting by various means has also been a part of certain religious rituals. For the bloodletter, letting blood by cutting is a catharsis. Bloodletting is also a catharsis for the one being cut. In addition to hopefully correcting an anatomical problem, and serving as a catharsis, surgery is a trauma causing the patient to take a time out in their life.

With all the tied-upness in the typical modern-day life, many people are trapped in the rat-race of life 24-7-365 with little downtime. Relationships, work, cellphone and computer use, driving, and all of the many challenges and stresses of life are non-stop. The resulting toxic energies get absorbed by the body. This absorbed energy causes muscles of the body to contract, shorten, stiffen, and tighten producing pain. The heart, stomach, and all of our muscles are likely targets of this pain.

The typical person confronted with pain may not allow themselves the downtime, rest, and proper self-care to heal and instead keeps up their regular pace. Undergoing surgery forces them to take downtime granting them much needed time off from work and physical rest. Perhaps certain elective surgeries might have the same outcome if performed by cutting anywhere. As long as vital structures are not cut, the main thing many elective surgeries may afford patients is the downtime necessary to rest and heal. Of course, this does not apply to those absolutely life-saving emergency and urgent surgeries including appendectomy, gallbladder removal, and similar surgeries.

Surgery has the effect of allowing the patient an extended downtime kind of like an extended Sabbath. Suddenly external stressors are minimized, and the patient can focus their energy on resting and healing. Chiropractic, acupuncture, and other therapies are similar in that they create a brief timeout, almost like a mini-Sabbath, during which, for the first time in their busy, stressful, day a patient may lie still without moving and feel the blood pulsing in their fingers and toes. Perhaps for some taking a vacation or extended timeout or adopting the religious Sabbath might be an excellent substitute for certain surgeries.

More:

Once upon a time there was a Temple in Jerusalem where people brought their first-born bulls, oxen, cows, goats, and sheep to be ritually sacrificed by the priests. This was a process of sensitizing the masses to be holy, G0dly, and kind. Instead of harming or killing themselves to kill their animal Soul, their first-born animals were killed. This was not senseless killing of animals with only a spiritual purpose. These animals also served as donations for the food of the priests.

The priests wore a set of special garments, washed their hands, and wielded a knife to perform the sacrifice killing the animal with a speedy painless technique. These animal sacrifices were discontinued with the destruction of the Temple in Jerusalem. Yet, nearly if not every day in every western country and city, there are certain people who, like the priests of old, don a special set of garments, ritually wash their hands, and

U R NOT WHAT U EAT

wield a knife to let blood. This bloodletting is done to people rather than animals. This is the practice of modern-day surgery occurring in hospitals and surgery centers. Perhaps all of modern-day surgeries are appropriate and necessary. Yet, perhaps some portion of these surgeries actually has the effect of allowing a sublimation of pain through the process of being surgically cut and then resting and healing. This sublimation is a therapeutic catharsis of individual and collective societal pain manifesting in both the surgeon and the patient. A portion of modern-day surgery may be serving the same purpose as the sacrifices of old.

22

The Soul Food Diet and Lifestyle for a New America

A dear friend once taught me the meaning of the word America in Hebrew. "Am" means nation, and "rica" means empty. America in Hebrew can mean a nation of emptiness. This emptiness would be a descriptive term similar to how the Jewish people might have been described while they were living in the desert after leaving Egypt. The desert was full of challenges which would all become clearer once the people received the Torah and its teachings regarding the path and process to connect with G0d and how to live a G0dly life as the Divine Soul.

A people living as their Divine Souls can best actualize themselves as human beings. "Human being" is a verb, and when we live as Divine Souls serving G0d and knowing what we are needed for rather than seeking to satisfy our needs, our "beingness" can become consistent thought, speech, and actions of lovingkindness. This pathway of actualizing our identities as Divine Souls, connecting to G0d, and being thought, speech, and actions of lovingkindness is the new Soul Food diet and lifestyle for a new America. It is the remedy for any sense of emptiness.

The most potent way any human being can impactfully change the world and America is by changing themselves. Power resides not with those who might be physically strong, accomplished, or monied with abundant possessions. Rather, it lies in the hands of those who can change themselves for the better. Let your "I" be the Divine Soul, and use your thought, speech, and action cautiously and wisely to connect with the Divine Ruler and other Divine Souls.

Recently we in America and humanity the world over have come face to face with a new enemy. The Coronavirus is forcing humankind (kind man) into relative isolation. We have entered our own relatively dark, silent, vulnerable, and separate sequestered "cocoons.". This process is reminiscent of a biblical disease called tzaraat in Hebrew. This disease was a spiritual disease with physical manifestations. It was so pervasive that it could affect all concentric layers beginning internally with the Soul, and progressing outward to include the body and skin, the clothes, and the house.

Although discussions and explanations of tzaraat focus on disease manifestations of the skin and hair, my own personal understanding is that the terms skin and hair are used symbolically to represent something of more profound significance. I believe the reference to the skin refers to the manifestation of the tzaraat disease in the "skins of the Soul." The skins of the Soul can be thought of as concentric layers enveloping the soul. These include the entire body, which is the first skin of the soul, the outer layer of which is the bodily skin itself. Then come the outer concentric layers of the clothes followed by the house.

I believe the biblical discussion of hair does not refer to our hair at all, but instead is meant to be symbolic. Just as there is almost no space between hairs and hairs cannot be counted, any hairbreadth of the body, as well as the clothes and house, could be involved with the disease. A comb is used to fashion hair, and to comb through the person's life would mean to analyze all of that person including soul, total body, and all connections and possessions leaving "no hair unturned."

Tzaraat resulted from having spiritually and physically separated one-self from G0d and one's Divine Soul identity and having instead found connection and meaning elsewhere. Tzaraat resulted from the prevalence of unclean thoughts, speech, and actions including those involving eating, relationships, business, and finding meaning and purpose in unclean endeavors. The flood of the earth in ancient time and the coronavirus of today may have a similar cause. The flood deprived all of mankind except for Noah and his family of the ability to make things right and heal. Thankfully, coronavirus, like tzaraat, is more forgiving and allows for healing.

Tzaraat was not the expertise of doctors, but instead was evaluated and treated by the priests of the time. Doctors, lawyers, and other professionals of today are biased by personal reward, profit motive, and financial gain, depending on what they do and how much they do. The priest was only biased to G0d and service of G0d and had no personal gain. Today's bias of personal gain could be significantly diminished or eliminated by putting doctors, lawyers, and other professionals on salary to eliminate the drive to do more for personal profit.

The priest evaluated every hairbreadth of your life, including Soul, body, life history, and all relationships, clothes, houses, and possessions. No hairbreadth of your life could be left unturned in searching for signs of the disease in your life. This procedure was unlike that of doctors and lawyers of today who spend little time, charge much, and often ignore essential life issues necessary to accurately identify and handle medical, legal, and other problems. Treatment involved separating from loved ones, connections, and possessions and going into isolation away from all of one's connections except for self and G0d. The priest would check on the sequestered individual each week until they showed signs of recovery after which they were permitted to return to the general population.

The goal of treatment of biblical tzaraat was that an imposed spiritual and physical separation in the face of a frightening disease would promote Soul searching and a return to G0d and Divine Soul self. This treatment might possibly be the best treatment for many people's problems today.

We encounter many medical, legal, social, financial, relationship, and other issues for which we visit all kinds of biased professionals who are tunnel vision trained and for which we get all sorts of treatments and services. Perhaps a better solution might be to take an extended time out and a period of separation to strengthen ourselves as Divine Souls and our connections with G0d. By doing so, our new perspective might shed light on our problems allowing us to realize the solutions, and our issues might even spontaneously disappear.

The priest as the "gatekeeper" for disease management with "managed care" based on the priest's lack of bias from profit motive and his role to search deeply and thoroughly through the patient's life, connections, and relationships is a suitable model for what managed healthcare could be today. This model would include not only making physicians salaried, but also training a layer of surgical specialists who do not operate, but instead evaluate patients for whether they might require surgery, or whether they may in fact recover without any surgery. This would allow many patients, who in the current system undergo surgery, to be treated successfully non-surgically. With this protective buffering layer, surgeons who actually operate could almost be on a surgical assembly line operating on patients who have been rigorously determined to require surgery. Incorporating these managed healthcare concepts could greatly reduce bias from profit motive.

Would our grandparents be more familiar with the "normal" pre-covid-19 coronavirus hustle and bustle way of life, or with the coronavirus mandated sequestered and "sheltered-in-place" lifestyle? All of the tech-nologies we have come to rely on, and that bring with them great stress and anxiety, were not around for our grandparents and are limited during isolation for coronavirus. They can readily take over our lives but living in isolation separated from others and from many technologies can create more freedom than before in many respects. This sense of freedom might be more recognizable to our grandparents, and so we might question which one of us is "normal" or more human and real? Are we more normal in the pre-coronavirus hustle and bustle state, or in the post-coronavirus quiet state?

When confronting a new problem, complaint, or sickness many patients present to their doctor with astonishment and ask, "I never had this before. Why should I have it now?" Every time I would hear this from a patient, I was struck by the underlying message this question implied. They were really and unrealistically saying that they didn't expect any life change, that aging and disease are not a reality, and we should be like robots, unchanging and fixed in time. But sometimes in life, "it is what it is," and certain things like aging and disease are unavoidable and bound to happen no matter what.

Since it is real and it is here, despite all the pain, suffering, tragedy, and death, we can make something worthwhile of the Coronavirus by using it as a wakeup call. We can interpret what we are going through as a struggle, trial, or test, and not a punishment of sickness and death. We can become awakened and inspired to become our Divine Soul identity and reach out to connect with G0d and others with lovingkindness. We can gather the strength to separate from and discontinue any toxic behaviors towards oneself and others. The lessons we learn in time of struggle and hardship can be used to build strength and courage for all time. In the short term, we can all spiritually transform into beautiful flying butterflies, and like the repetitive molting of the lobster, continue to repeat this process over and over throughout our lives. By positively transforming ourselves we will positively and impactfully change America and the world for the better.

More:

There was a poor man who had a wife and seven young children, all of whom lived in a one-room apartment. He and his wife were frequently arguing due to their cramped quarters and limited funds to advance in life. It was always very hectic, and he was very sad that he could not create a better situation for his family. He went to the respected elder wise man of the town and asked for advice. He told him to bring a live chicken into the apartment. When he went home and told his wife what the wise man said, she couldn't understand it. But they both respected him, so he brought a chicken into the apartment.

Sometime later things were more hectic, so he again visited the wise man and explained that the situation was worse than before. The wise man reassured him and told him to bring a goat into his apartment. Again, he returned to his wife and shared the wise man's advice. They were both perplexed, but he listened to the wise man and brought a goat into their apartment. The resultant commotion was unbearable.

The family put up with this horrible situation for a while until he again presented to the wise man asking for help. This time he was told to bring a donkey into the apartment. He tried to explain to the wise man how impossible that was, but the wise man insisted. So he brought a donkey home to the apartment and from then on it was pure pandemonium. After some time, he returned to the wise man and said that he, his wife, and his children were at their wits' end. None of the recommendations he implemented so far were helpful.

The wise man told him to now remove the chicken, goat, and donkey from their apartment. When he did that, leaving only him, his wife, and their children, everything suddenly seemed so peaceful. Back to their original situation which previously was intolerable, now they were overjoyed. Their disheartened attitude about their situation was miraculously transformed to one of happiness. The lesson from this story is that there may be times in life that things may seem unbearable, yet all that may be needed to fix the problem is a change in perspective and attitude. With the right wisdom, lifestyle diet, and toolbox any pain can be transformed to pearls of wisdom and joy.

www.ingramcontent.com/pod-product-compliance
Lightning Source LLC
Chambersburg PA
CBHW051025030426
42336CB00015B/2725